I0428921

SUPER HEALTHY SMOOTHIES

A Well Balanced Smoothie System for Wellness, Detox, Diet & Energy

JONATHAN HALPERN, PhD

Copyright © 2016 Jonathan Halpern

All rights reserved.

ISBN-10: 1532784600
ISBN-13: 978-1532784606

Without limiting the rights under copyright reserved above, no part of this publication may be reproduced, stored in or introduced into a retrieval system, or transmitted in any form or by any means (electronic, mechanical, photocopying, recording, scanning, or otherwise), without the prior written permission of the copyright owner of this book. The scanning, duplication and distribution of this book via the Internet, or via any other means without permission of the author is illegal and punishable by law. Please purchase only authorized electronic editions, and do not participate in or encourage electronic piracy. Thank you.

DEDICATION

This is for you, mom. Thank you for testing my smoothie recipes and finding simple and effective ways to make them much better. Thank you for always being there for us in so many ways.

ACKNOWLEDGMENT

Thanks to Lindsay Kilminster for cover graphics design.

DISCLAIMER AND LEGAL NOTICES

All content ("content"), including text, graphics, images and information available on or through this publication are for general informational purposes only. It is not designed to, and does not provide medical or technical advice. By providing the information contained herein we are not diagnosing, treating, curing, mitigating, or preventing any type of disease, disorder or medical condition. If advice concerning medical, technical, nutritional, well-being or related matters is needed, the services of a fully qualified and licensed professional should be sought. It is advisable to seek the advice of a licensed healthcare professional before starting any type of health related treatment regimen. Never disregard professional medical or technical advice, or delay in seeking it, because of something you have read on or through this publication. Never rely on information available on or through this publication in place of seeking professional medical or technical advice.

The writer and publisher of this publication are not responsible or liable for any advice, course of treatment, diagnosis, analysis or any other information, services or products that you obtain through this publication. You are encouraged to confer with your doctor and technical and legal experts with regard to information contained on or through this publication. After reading information available on or through this publication, you are encouraged to review the information carefully with your professional health care provider, legal and technical professionals. You should be aware of any laws, which govern medical, legal and technical practices in your country and state.

The information presented herein only represents the view of the author at the date of publication. Because of the rapid rate with which various conditions change, the author reserves the right to alter, modify and update his opinion and the content of this publication in accordance with the new conditions as he perceives them. While every attempt has been made to verify the information provided in this publication, neither the author nor the publisher assume any responsibility for errors, inaccuracies or omissions. You are encouraged to confer with your doctor and technical experts with regard to information contained on or through this publication. After reading information available on or through this publication, you are encouraged to review the information carefully with your professional health care provider and technical professionals.

Any slights of individuals or organizations are unintentional. Any reference to any person or business whether living or dead is purely coincidental.

TABLE OF CONTENTS

INTRODUCTION

I first became interested in making smoothies years ago when I was working on my PhD in health sciences and looking for a quick and easy method to boost and balance my nutrition while accommodating a busy lifestyle. I found making smoothies a very effective way to integrate the principles of modern nutrition science, alternative and complementary medicine and traditional medicine. Over time, with changing seasons, needs and conditions – I modified, improved and simplified the recipes and then started making smoothies for friends and relatives, incorporating their useful feedback and requests where possible. Gradually, a nice smoothie system evolved. When friends started asking me how to actually make these smoothies I decided to put it all together in a book with detailed recipes and clear instructions to ensure consistently good results. Please feel free to send me your feedback and suggestions for future editions.

This book is for you if you want to -

- Improve your well-being
- Feel lighter and more energized
- Make dieting easier
- Save time and money
- Learn about food and health

About the smoothie recipes in this book:

- Super healthy, low calorie, detoxing, energizing

- Quick, easy and tasty

- Nutritionally, seasonally and energetically balanced

- Accommodate a wide range of diets, needs and activity levels

- Combinations of smoothies, juices and teas

- Include a detailed list of ingredient substitutions

- Include detailed smoothie texture control methods

Additional useful information including:

- Detailed information on all the ingredients

- Comparison between smoothies, juices and salads

- Foundation nutritional knowledge for balanced smoothies

- Foundation energetic knowledge for balanced smoothies

- Adapting smoothies to changing needs and conditions

- Adapting smoothies to different types of diets

- Information on blenders and other required tools

- Information about organic, non-organic and GMO food

WHY SMOOTHIE?

In a nutshell

1. Smoothies are a simple and effective way to ensure you consume adequate levels of fresh vegetables and fruit, vitamins, minerals, antioxidants, electrolytes, oils, fiber and a range of other important phyto-nutrients.

2. Smoothies help increase water and fiber intake and contribute to improved hydration and better regulation of bowel movements.

3. Smoothies are a great way to have a meal on the go without gulping down food that has not been chewed properly.

4. Smoothies are refreshing and nutritious but light and easy to digest to help you feel energized, light and able to function better.

5. Smoothies save time. Preparing a nice smoothie is faster than preparing a meal. Consuming a smoothie is much faster than chewing a meal.

6. Smoothies are filling and satisfying and can help in maintaining diets, losing weight and keeping it off with less food cravings and unbalanced appetite.

7. Kids love smoothies and by adding a higher proportion of fruit you can make the smoothies more attractive to kids' sweet palates. Some kids don't like chewing raw veggies but

they usually love the texture of smoothies.

Smoothies v Juicing

Some are big fans of smoothies where as others prefer juicing. So which is better? The simple answer is that both smoothies and juices are excellent health promoting tools. Both enable consuming higher amounts of nutrients and are easy to digest. However, there are several important differences between smoothies and juices that should be pointed out.

Nutritional content – smoothies v juices

Smoothies are a whole food made by blending vegetables and/or fruit mixed with liquids. The nutritional content is retained fully in a liquefied easier to digest form. On the other hand, juices are made by extracting the liquid content of veggies and/or fruit. The water content of fruit and vegetables ranges from 79 percent to 96 percent. That leaves 11 to 4 percent leftover pulp containing mostly fiber but also some nutrients.

The amount of nutrients and fiber lost in the juicing process depends on the type of fruit/vegetables and the type of juicer being used. Powerful more expensive juicers are able to extract more nutrients, especially from skins of fruit/vegetables. However, regardless of the juicer being used, most of the fiber is lost unless you keep the pulp and use it for making soups or other dishes.

The quality of the blender used to make the smoothie may also make a difference in nutrient bio-availability. Finer particles result in higher bio-availability and ease of digestion.

Nutrient bio-availability– smoothies v juices

Nutrient bio-availability may decrease as a result of heat and oxidation generated during the juicing or blending process. These effects are specific to blender or juicer models. Some juicers use slow extraction to maintain lower temperatures. In general mineral bio-availability is only slightly lower in smoothies compared to juices. On the other hand, vitamin C and A content may be significantly higher in juices compared to smoothies (up to 100 percent higher). However, this is offset by a much higher content of both non-soluble and soluble fibers in smoothies.

Ease of digestion – smoothies v juices

Fruit and vegetable juices are easier to digest and considered highly concentrated bio-available foods. Digesting juices requires very little bio-energy. And as mentioned above the bio-availability of nutrients in juices is higher. For people with extremely compromised digestive systems and/or very weakened constitutions juices provide an advantage. However, the ease of digestion and nutrient bio-availability of smoothies is still much higher than that of most other foods. Furthermore, smoothies like juices do not require chewing.

Glycemic index (GI) – smoothies v juices

Glycemic index (GI) indicates the effect of a food on blood glucose level. The higher the index, the faster the rise in blood glucose level after consumption of a particular food. Pure glucose has the highest

GI of 100. In general, if you compare smoothies to juices that are prepared using similar ingredients then the smoothies would have a lower GI than juices because the fiber and oil content slows down the absorption of sugars into the bloodstream. This is an important point to remember for anyone who is suffering from diabetes or classified by their health practitioner as "pre-diabetic" or as having the "metabolic syndrome". However, the GI of juices can also be lowered significantly but reducing to a minimum the amounts of sweet fruits (such as oranges, grapes etc.) and sweet vegetables (such as beets, carrots etc.). It is worth mentioning that lemons and avocados, two nutrient dense foods classified as fruits, have very low GI. I recommend using both in many smoothie recipes.

Appetite control and diet support – smoothies v juices

Smoothies are more filling than juices because of their fiber and oil content. Overall smoothies are more filling than juices, slow down digestion, and are more effective in delaying hunger onset. For the same type and quantity of ingredients, juices have a higher level of sugar. This may result in more rapid and stronger stimulation of the digestive system and earlier hunger onset. Depending on the ingredients, a smoothie can serve as a complete meal. Compared to juices, smoothies cause lower sugar level spikes and keeps you full much longer. That may help you reduce food cravings and calorie consumption in a painless and healthy way without having to resort to extreme diets (or worse – diet pills).

Cost of smoothies v juices

In general, the cost per cup of smoothie is lower than the cost per cup of juice when using similar ingredients. There are two reasons for this: First – juicing results in loss of fiber. Second – smoothies are made by blending fruit and vegetables with about 20 percent (in volume) of added liquids. Bottom line – smoothies provide a greater volume when using the same amount of raw ingredients.

Time saving smoothies v juices

Making a smoothie usually takes less time than juicing. When making a smoothie, all the chopped ingredients go into the blender jug together and within a minute of pressing a button the smoothie is ready to be served. Juicing is usually a more elaborate process as the chopped ingredients need to be inserted manually one by one. Furthermore, cleaning a juicer usually takes longer. There are more parts that need to be uninstalled, washed, dried and put together again.

Smoothies vs salads

It is nice to have a salad with your meal or on its own. Chewing mindfully enhances the experience and gives a better opportunity to enjoy the flavors and textures of the food. If you happen to be an omnivore, having a green salad together with animal based foods makes sense because it may help counteract some of the negative side effects of eating cooked animal proteins (e.g. eggs, fish, chicken, beef) by providing the fiber lacking in these foods and also by helping detoxify some of the undesirable byproducts of cooking these foods in high temperatures. However, smoothies have their own advantages as pointed out below.

Digestion and assimilation – smoothies v salads

We have teeth for a reason. Most meals should probably be done sitting down peacefully, eating mindfully and chewing well. Chewing is an important part of the digestive process as it breaks food into small particles that are easier to digest. Natural health proponents recommend chewing food thoroughly until the food is liquefied in order to improve digestion and absorption of nutrients and prevent partially digested food from entering the blood stream as this may trigger allergic reactions and other adverse effects.

Chewing also mixes the food with saliva that acts as a lubricant that helps the food slide down the esophagus. Saliva contains antibacterial and acidity regulating compounds and enzymes. The main enzymes are salivary amylase (also called ptyalin) and salivary lipase. These start the process of digesting starches and fats respectively. The process is continued by digestive enzymes produced by the pancreas and secreted into the duodenum which is the first section of the small intestine.

Research has shown that eating in a hurry and gulping down the food increases stress levels and activates the sympathetic nervous system. Unfortunately, most people do not have the patience to chew their food well. We live in a fast paced world where many people have their meals while using their smart phones and other mobile devices.

This makes it harder to relax and chew well. Therefore, if you don't have the time or patience to sit down quietly for a meal, then having a smoothie is preferable to eating fast and gulping the food without chewing it well.

The smoothie blending process breaks down the raw food and mixes it thoroughly with water and oils. When using a good quality blender, the resulting mixture contains very small particles. In fact, smaller than what is achieved by chewing well. The liquid component helps absorb a higher proportion of water soluble nutrients. The oil component helps absorb a higher proportion of fat soluble nutrients. The digestive process requires significant amounts of bio-energy. By blending and liquefying the food well, much of this energy is saved and can be utilized for other important tasks such as detoxifying, body maintenance and repair. When having your smoothie, it is preferable to consume it slowly as if eating solid food, using a spoon rather than gulping it down. This slows down the process and allows the smoothie to mix with saliva. It is also more enjoyable.

Overall nutrient intake – smoothies v salads

Smoothies allow increasing your nutrient and fiber intake compared to salads. Blending compacts a substantial volume of vegetables and fruit to fit into a small bowl or mug. You can then mix additional oils, supplements and super foods such chlorella powder, spirulina powder or wheat-grass powder or protein powder concentrate. You can also grind some seeds and mix them into your smoothie. Overall, these synergistic methods turn the smoothie into a concentrated nutrient dense easy to digest super food. These will be discussed in detail in following sections.

Time saving smoothies v salads

Compared to salads – smoothies allow consuming a greater and more diverse nutritional profile without having to sit down for a meal and do much chewing. That saves time! Less dishes to clean too!

FOUNDATIONS OF HEALTHY SMOOTHIES

In a nutshell

To get the most out of our smoothies and maximize health benefits we need to use these important principles:

- **Balanced and optimized nutrition**
- **Alkaline-acid balance**
- **Antioxidant balance**
- **Electrolyte balance**
- **Fatty Acid balance**
- **Protein balance**
- **Fiber balance**
- **Gut microbiome balance**
- **Energetic balance**
- **Seasonal balance**
- **Holistic balance**

Note:

The following sections explain how these principles are applied in the super healthy balanced smoothies.

Balanced and optimized nutrition

In general, there are two important processes related to diet and nutrition. One side of the equation includes digestion and absorption and the other side includes elimination and detoxification. To maintain a state of optimal health the equation needs to be balanced. Both sides of the equation require energy and draw on the body's resources. If the equation becomes imbalanced towards one side it usually results in the other side performing below par. For example, a diet that is too rich in carbohydrates and/or proteins and/or fats may tax the digestive system and hinder elimination and detoxification. This may result in accumulation of phlegm and toxins in the body. On the other hand, a detox diet that provides only minimal amounts of nutrients, may provide short term benefits by assisting detoxification and elimination but if continued unsupervised for a long time it may result in depletion, weakness and damage to organs. The balanced smoothie aims at boosting both sides of the equation by maximizing nutrition while minimizing energy expenditure and allowing better detoxification.

There are diverse opinions as to what constitutes a super-food. Some scientists and nutritionists are of the opinion that there is no such thing as a super-food and that the term is nothing but a marketing gimmick designed to promote expensive supplements. Indeed, the market is flooded with expensive supplements and packaged health-food products claiming a range of health benefits. Often these claims are not backed by scientific evidence and may add a financial burden to existing health and emotional concerns. Perhaps a good way is to describe a super-food is a nutrient dense easy to digest food providing large amounts of essentials nutrients (e.g. antioxidants vitamins, minerals, fatty acids, amino acids). This is best achieved by a synergistic combination of foods working together as a team as put into practice in the core balanced smoothie recipe

The core balanced smoothie balances food categories, colors, flavors and energies. It aims at creating a synergistic "team" of foods that complement each other and work together to achieve optimal concentrated nutrition including natural anti-inflammatory and antioxidant phyto-nutrients, electrolytes, enzymes, vitamins, minerals, a good ratio of omega-3 to omega-6 polyunsaturated fatty acids, mono-unsaturated fatty acids, small amounts of plant based "complete" protein with all essential amino acids, soluble and non-soluble fibers and pre-biotics and other important phyto-nutrients. The core balanced smoothie recipe provides optimized nutritional content by including foods from these categories:

Green leafy vegetables (e.g. kale, spinach, beet greens, sweet potato greens)

Other vegetables (e.g. tomatoes, cucumbers, capsicums)

Sprouts (e.g. broccoli, alfalfa, radish & onion sprouts)

Low sugar fruits (e.g. lemons, limes, berries)

Small amounts of seeds (e.g. chia seeds, flaxseeds, black nigella seeds, pumpkin)

Seaweed (e.g. dried nori seaweed)

Oils (e.g. olive oil, coconut oil)

Condiments (e.g. apple cider vinegar, pickled ginger, pickled beetroot)

Spices (e.g. ginger, cinnamon, turmeric, black pepper)

Fibers (e.g. psyllium seed husk, coconut flour)

Liquids and juices (e.g. coconut water, pomegranate juice, beetroot juice, aloe Vera juice)

Supplements – optional (e.g. spirulina, chlorella, wheatgrass powder, barley grass powder, whey protein concentrate powder, full spectrum vegan protein concentrate)

The core balanced recipe is not intended as a complete meal on its own as it is relatively low on protein. In order to build protein, the body requires adequate amounts of nine essential amino acids that must come from food in specific proportions. These are Histamine, Isoleucine, Leucine, Lysine, Methionine, Phenylalanine, Threonine, Tryptophan and Valine. A food containing all these nine essential amino acids in the right proportions is called "complete" protein. Supplements with high concentrations of complete protein are chlorella powder and spirulina powder. However, they are relatively expensive and have a strong flavor so are usually consumed in small amounts. To boost your smoothie and transform it into a complete meal you would need to add a scoop of full spectrum protein concentrate powder. If you are not a vegan and not allergic/sensitive to dairy products, you can add a scoop of whey protein concentrate powder. If you are vegan or allergic/sensitive to dairy products, you can add a scoop of full spectrum vegan protein powder. The good brands usually have a mix of several plant based protein concentrates such as chia seed protein, hemp seed protein, pea protein and potato protein.

Alkaline-acid balance

An important health principle is maintaining the alkaline/acid balance in the body. All foods are either acidic, alkaline or neutral in nature. Acidity and alkalinity of water soluble substances is measured using the pH scale ranging from 1 to 14 with 1 indicating extremely acidic, 14 extremely alkaline and 7 located mid-scale (i.e. neutral). Distilled water is always neutral with a pH of 7.

The pH of normal human blood is tightly regulated by the body between 7.35 and 7.45 (slightly alkaline). Different health conditions and also ingested foods may alter the acid/alkaline balance and even slight changes may have a detrimental effect on our health. Different sections of the digestive system are regulated and maintained at specific pH levels by secretions along the digestive tract. Undiluted stomach gastric juices have a pH of 2-3. This changes to about pH 6 in the duodenum, pH 7.4 in the terminal ileum, pH 5.7 in the cecum and pH 6.7 in the rectum. Stomach weakness may lead to decreased secretion of gastric juices, reduced acidity levels, poor digestion and even malnutrition. By the same token, very acidic conditions in the intestines may cause an imbalance in intestinal microbiome leading to a host of health problems such as allergies, flatulence, diarrhea, constipation or far worse.

Life style affects the acid/alkaline balance. A poor diet, lack of sleep, prolonged stress, lack of exercise or over-exercise without adequate recovery may result in elevated acidity levels. Shallow breathing and poor posture may also reduce the body's efficiency in getting rid of carbon-dioxide leading to increased blood acidity levels.

The modern western diet with a lot of meat, sugars, grains and processed carbohydrates is imbalanced towards acid forming foods and tends to acidify the body. A chronic tendency towards acidity in the blood and tissues is thought to increase the risk of a range of health conditions. In an attempt to reduce acidity level, the body is forced to draw upon its mineral reserves. Most calcium reserves are stored in the bones so this may eventually lead to weakening of the bones, osteopenia or even osteoporosis especially in post-menopausal women but also in older men. Falls that lead to hip and spinal fractures are one of the leading causes of loss of mobility, loss of independence and even premature death among the elderly population. Therefore, maintaining a more alkaline diet may contribute to wellness and longevity.

Various diets and supplements have been developed to help regulate the body's alkaline/acid balance. To balance overall acidic tendencies in the body it is recommended to significantly increase the intake of vegetables and fruit and at the same time decrease the intake of acid forming foods such as sugars, most grains, processed carbohydrates of all types and meat.

An acidic food doesn't necessarily make the blood more acidic and vice versa. For example, lemon juice is acidic (pH of about 2) but has an alkalizing effect on the body. On the other hand, white sugar is not acidic but has an acidifying effect on the body.

The core balanced smoothie recipe incorporates a range of alkalizing vegetables and condiments (e.g. green leafy vegetables, cucumbers, celery, spirulina, chlorella, wheatgrass and barley green powders, seaweed, Celtic sea salt or Himalayan salt) and small quantities of nutrient dense alkaline forming fruit that are low on sugar (e.g. berries, lemons, limes, kiwis) together with oils and seeds that synergistically enhance nutrient absorption from all other ingredients. The result is optimized intake of large quantities of phytonutrients and organic minerals that help alkalize the body.

Antioxidant Balance

Antioxidants are molecules that inhibit oxidation of other molecules. Oxidation is a natural process in all living organisms and in the human body it plays an important role in energy production and in fighting invading pathogens. However, oxidation may produce free radicals, and if excessive may damage cells. Antioxidants can help stop these destructive oxidation chain reactions.

Many studies have shown that antioxidants may play an important role in the reducing the risk of heart disease, cancer, Alzheimer's, Parkinson's and a range of other conditions.

Living organisms use many types of antioxidants – some important antioxidants such as glutathione are produced internally and some obtained through the diet. Antioxidant content is measured and quantified in the lab using "Oxygen Radical Absorbency Capacity" (ORAC). Among available foods, some of the highest on the ORAC scale are spices (e.g. cloves, cinnamon, turmeric), cocoa products (e.g. dark cocoa and dark chocolate), berries (e.g. goji berries, blueberries, elderberries, blackberries, strawberries), some nuts (e.g. pecans), some seeds (e.g. chia), some green leafy vegetables (e.g. kale). However, it is worth pointing out that a high ORAC doesn't necessarily translate to high antioxidant activity inside the body ("in vivo").

Each antioxidant has its own unique way of working so loading up on a particular antioxidant (e.g. vitamin C) may not necessarily produce the desired outcomes. Consuming large amounts of antioxidants in the form of supplements may provide both advantages and disadvantage and should only be prescribed by a health practitioner. For most people, the best way to get a wide range of antioxidants is to consume fresh vegetables, fruit, seeds and beans that have violet, purple, blue, green, yellow, orange, red colors, or more simply – all the colors of the rainbow.

The balanced smoothie provides a wide range of antioxidants from green leafy vegetables, lemons and limes, berries, chia and flax seeds to name a few. Some of the important antioxidants belong to classes of molecules called carotenoids and flavonoids. Table 1 below lists colorful antioxidants and the foods that are rich in these important phytonutrients.

Table 1 – Antioxidants in foods

Foods	Antioxidant	Class	Color
leafy greens (e.g. spinach, kale), peas, broccoli, celery, corn, wolfberries, saffron,	Lutein, Zeaxanthin, *Meso-zeaxanthin*	carotenoids	yellow, green
Turmeric	Curcumin	Curcuminoides	yellow
oranges, tangerines, papaws, carrots, peaches, apricots, spinach and cantaloupe, pumpkin	Beta-Carotene, Alpha-carotene, Cryptoxanthin	carotenoids	orange
Tomatoes, strawberries, goji berries, raspberries, cherries, pomegranate, beets, red cabbage, chili, watermelon and pink grapefruit	Lycopene	carotenoids	red
Red peppers	Capasanthin, capsorubin	carotenoids	red
Blueberries	Anthocyanins	Flavonoids	Blue, purple, violet

Electrolyte balance

Electrolytes are substances that when dissolved in water separate into positive and negative ions (cations and anions) and enable conduction of electric currents. The main electrolyte ions are sodium ($Na+$), potassium ($K+$), calcium ($Ca^{2}+$), magnesium($Mg^{2}+$), chloride ($Cl-$), hydrogen phosphate ($HPO_4{}^{2}-$), and hydrogen carbonate (HCO_3-). Electrolytes are essential for enabling bio-electric currents that relay signals from the brain and nervous system to the skin, muscles, heart and other organs and back to the brain. Electrolytes are also involved in maintaining correct blood and cellular acid – alkaline (pH) balance.

We lose electrolytes via sweating and urination especially during hot weather and sports activity. Sodium is the most depleted electrolyte followed by potassium. We need to replenish lost electrolytes in order to maintain a state of good hydration and good health. Drinking water may not be enough as most water sources provide only very small amounts of these electrolytes, filtered reverse osmosis water only provides tiny amounts (most mineral content is lost during the filtration process) and distilled water has none. On the other hand, coconut water is a rich in potassium, sodium, magnesium, calcium and phosphorous and is a well-balanced natural source of electrolytes. Coconut water works very well as the liquid base for the balanced sports smoothie.

The balanced smoothie naturally contains significant amounts of electrolytes and by adding coconut water and slightly more sea salt you can boost the smoothie's electrolytes levels further resulting in a formula that is more natural, hydrating and alkalizing than most commercially available sports drinks, yet does not contain artificial sweeteners, preservatives, colors, caffeine and commercial sugars that acidify and overstimulate the and may cause blood sugar level spikes followed by insulin level spikes. The caffeine in some sports drinks may actually have a diuretic effect leading to dehydration and thus defeating the purpose.

Notes:

1. Some vegetables such as celery, parsley and beets have a mild diuretic affect. However, the balanced smoothie only includes moderate amounts of these very healthy and nutritious veggies.
2. Vegetable juices may produce a greater diuretic effect than smoothies (having similar ingredients) due to their much lower fiber and oil content that results in a more rapid absorption and excretion.

Fatty acids balance

This is a very important topic but beyond the scope of this book so will only be mentioned here briefly. Omega 3, 6, 7 and 9 are a group of essential unsaturated fatty acids. They cannot be produced by the body and must be derived from food. Omega-3 fatty acids play an important role in maintaining the health of the heart, brain, blood vessels and joints. They may help prevent inflammation, auto-immune diseases and even cancer. The three main types of Omega-3 fatty acids are:

ALA (alpha-linolenic acid) found in a range of plant food sources such as flaxseed, chia seed, and walnuts.

EPA (eicosapentaenoic acid) found mainly in fish and shellfish.

DHA (docosahexaenoic acid) found mainly in fish, shellfish and some seaweed and algae.

The human body is able to convert ALA into EPA but not very efficiently. The conversion of ALA into DHA is very inefficient and requires large amounts of ALA. Recent studies have led scientists to believe that consumption of large amounts of ALA may be detrimental to our health. Since both EPA and DHA are very important for maintaining our health it is essential that we consume them either by eating fish and/or shellfish or by taking supplements (e.g. krill oil or fish oil). However, consuming moderate amounts of ALA from plant based sources does have important health benefits such as helping regulate blood sugar levels.

The ideal ratio between Omega-3 and Omega-6 fatty acids is about 1:1 (i.e. in equal proportion) and had been maintained by our ancestors for millennia. The modern western diet contain too much Omega-6 and too little Omega-3 fatty acids with a ratio of Omega-3 to Omega-6 may anywhere between 1:20 to 1:50. Scientists believe that this extreme Omega-3 to 6 imbalance predisposes the body to a range of health disorders that have increased in modern times.

The main causes for Omega-3 to Omega-6 imbalance at present are the wide spread use of Omega-6 rich vegetable oils (including most vegetable oil blends, corn, soy, safflower, sunflower and sesame oils) and the decreasing amounts of fish in the diet. Even if you don't use Omega-6 oils for cooking you may still be exposed to them when consuming a wide range of processed foods. A step in the right direction would be to reduce consumption of processed foods, eliminate vegetable oils (except for olive oil and coconut oil) and introduce the balanced smoothie on a daily basis.

The core balanced smoothie provides small amounts of fatty acids with a good ratio of omega-3 to omega-6 fatty acids with the Chia seeds and flaxseed providing plant based omega-3 fatty acids.

The core balanced smoothie also provides mono-unsaturated fatty acids (MUFA) from olive oil and avocado that have both been shown to improve blood cholesterol and lipid profile. They are low on Omega-6 fatty acids so do not have a substantial effect on the Omega 3 to 6 balance and also enhance absorption and assimilation of fat soluble phyto-nutrients such as lutein and carotene, including pro-vitamin A carotenoid.

If room temperature is above 24 degrees Celsius (75 degrees Fahrenheit) coconut oil may also added providing medium-chain saturated fatty acids (MCFA). At lower temperatures, coconut oil solidifies and is not suitable for making smoothies. Coconut oil has been shown to improve blood cholesterol and lipid profile and is also anti-bacterial, anti-fungal and anti-parasitic. It also enhances absorption and assimilation of fat soluble phyto-nutrients such as lutein and carotene including pro-vitamin A carotenoid.

Protein balance

The body builds proteins from basic building blocks called amino acids. These are divided into essential, conditionally essential and non-essential amino acids. The essential amino acids cannot be synthesized by the body and must come from food. Non-essential amino acids can be synthesized by the body and conditionally essential amino acids can be synthesized by the body under normal conditions in healthy people. In order to synthesize protein, the body needs an adequate supply of all the essential amino acids in the right proportions. A food source that satisfies this requirement is considered to be a "complete protein".

Proteins from animal sources are complete proteins. Many plant proteins are not "complete proteins" although some are (e.g. soybeans, chia seeds, hemp seeds, quinoa seeds and spirulina). When using plant sources that do not have "complete proteins" we need to combine complementary foods. For example – whole grains and legumes or legumes and seeds. However, some people have difficulty digesting substantial amounts of nuts, seeds or even legumes. Others are sensitive to grains or gluten intolerant. So finding a suitable complete protein combination may be challenging for some people.

The core balanced smoothie recipe is not intended to serve as a complete meal on its own. It includes small amounts of chia seeds, spirulina and chlorella that are excellent sources of "complete" vegan protein but these are relatively small. In order to boost the smoothie to provide substantial amounts of "complete" protein you can add a scoop of whey protein concentrate powder or a scoop of "full spectrum" vegan protein concentrate powder.

Fiber balance

There are two types of fibers, namely insoluble and soluble fibers. Insoluble fibers include cellulose, hemicelluloses and lignins. Soluble fibers include pectins, gums and mucilage. Insoluble fiber is found in the skins of fruit and vegetables and in the bran of whole grains. Soluble fiber can be found in some vegetables, fruit and legumes, psyllium seed husks and other seed husks (e.g. chia and flaxseed).

Insoluble fibers play a very important role in digestive health by adding bulk to feces, speeding the passage of food via the digestive tract, helping prevent constipation, promoting regularity and supporting easier elimination. Easier and faster passage of food via the digestive tract may help in reducing fermentation and putrefaction, maintaining a healthy balanced microbiota and reducing the risk of a range of health problems from hemorrhoids to bowel cancer. The importance of insoluble dietary fiber is even greater in omnivore diets and some vegetarian diets that contain foods from animal sources that are lacking in fiber.

Soluble fiber tends to absorb water, swell and become sticky, mucilaginous or gel like. This may help slow digestion of food and contribute to a feeling of fullness and satiety for longer periods. It may also help control blood cholesterol and blood glucose levels and help manage both diarrhea and loose stools.

Soluble fibers are considered a pre-biotic, serving as a food source for the good bacteria (probiotics) that reside in the human gut.

The core balanced smoothie recipe contains ample amounts of soluble and insoluble fibers. Green leafy vegetables are rich in insoluble fiber. Chia and flax seeds are rich in soluble fiber. You can boost the soluble fiber content by adding one teaspoon of psyllium seed husks or coconut flour or shredded citrus rind.

Notes:

1. Remember – everything in moderation! Consuming too much fiber may result in reduced nutrient absorption, lose stools, bloating and even flatulence although the latter is often the result of too much fruit in the smoothie or having the smoothie right after having a big meal. Always try to have your smoothies 1-2 hours at least before having a meal to allow digestion and free passage of sugars and other fermentable foods. I try to have my smoothie in the morning and my other meal(s) later in the day.

2. Coconut flour is very rich in fiber but should be used in small quantities (1-2 tsp) to prevent flatulence and discomfort.

Gut microbiome balance

Gut health, effective nutrient absorption and detoxification all depend on a well-balanced and healthy gut microbiome (also called microbiota) consisting of the trillions of microorganisms living in the digestive tract. The huge microbiome in the gut includes the good guys (i.e. probiotics), the bad guys (such as a potentially nasty yeast called candida albicans) and lots of other benign - "neutral" residents. The probiotics play an important role in breaking down and metabolizing food and also in neutralizing food based toxins. Scientists believe that healthy gut microbiota can produce substantial amounts of vitamin K2 and several B group vitamins, including Biotin and Folate. Some food related lactic acid bacteria (LAB) may even be able to produce cobalamin (vitamin B12).

Individuals may have diverse gut microbiota due to their diets and exposure to toxins and medications. Antibiotics have an adverse effect on gut microbiota. These include prescription antibiotics and also antibiotics consumed by eating (non-organic) meat, dairy products and eggs of farmed animals that had been treated with antibiotics against infections or for stimulating growth.
To control the "bad" guys living in gut, we need to restrict our consumption of sugars and processed foods. To help the "good" guys (probiotics) we need to consume the foods they thrive on. An important component of probiotic supporting food is called prebiotics and it consists mainly of fibers of fruit, vegetables, nuts and seeds.

The core balanced smoothie recipe includes lots of good sources of prebiotic fiber from green leafy vegetables, small amount of fruit, chia and flaxseeds. By adding psyllium seed husks and coconut flour you can further boost the prebiotic power of your smoothie.

Note:

Remember – everything in moderation! Consuming too much prebiotic fiber may result in reduced nutrient absorption, lose stools, bloating and even flatulence.

Food Energetics

Traditional Medicine maintains that each vegetable, fruit, herb and mineral has unique energetic properties including energy level, energy flow direction and the systems in the body it affects most.

Energy level

Any food may have one of the following energy levels: hot, warm, neutral, cool, cold. Cooked foods especially meat (if you are an omnivore) are energetically much warmer than fruit and vegetables that form the bulk of raw smoothies. The core balanced smoothie recipe contains ingredients with various energy levels that balance each other out:

> **Cool –** Green leafy veggies, cucumbers, cabbage, sprouts, lemons and limes are cooling
>
> **Neutral –** Berries, beetroot, pomegranates and seeds are neutral
>
> **Warm –** Pickled ginger, turmeric, vinegar, citrus peels, basil, coconut and olive oil are warm
>
> **Hot -**Black pepper, ginger powder, cinnamon powder and chilies heat up the digestive system and other organs.

Table 2 below lists smoothies ingredients and their energetic level.

Table 2 – Foods and their energetic levels

Energy	Examples of smoothie ingredients
hot	Chilies, black pepper, cinnamon, dried ginger,
warm	Fresh ginger, garlic, onions, leeks, dates, guava, pawpaw, ripe citrus peels, spearmint, basil, vinegar, coconut, coffee, pawpaw seeds, coconut oil, olive oil, turmeric
neutral	Goji berries, pawpaw, grapes, plums, apricots, tomatoes, carrots, avocado, beetroot, pomegranates, carrot, raw cocoa, mango, pawpaw, pineapple, cherry, most seeds
cool	Most green leafy veg, celery, cucumber, alfalfa sprouts, lettuce, cabbage, tomato, kiwi, most melons, water melon, peeled citrus fruits, pear, apple, pomegranate, banana strawberries, green tea, Peppermint, nori seaweed
cold	Kelp, some green teas

Notes:

1. Hot spices such as black pepper, ginger and cinnamon powders are only used in very small amounts to balance out much larger amounts of cool ingredients. Neutral ingredients do not need balancing out.

2. Hot spices and pickled ginger are only be used sparingly so as not to make the smoothies too spicy. Everything in

moderation! Remember – smoothies are just part of your diet and may help balance out foods that are much warmer energetically and vice versa.

Energy flow

Each food may affect body energy flow direction in one of the following ways:

1. supporting downward energy flow
2. supporting upward energy flow
3. supporting inward energy flow
4. supporting outward energy flow
5. neutral effect

The core balanced smoothie recipe contains ingredients with various energy flow properties and they tend to balance each other out:

upward – sprouts, some leafy greens – have upward flowing energy

downward – peeled ginger, turmeric, salt, carrots – downward flowing energy

inward -vinegar, seeds – concentrating inward flowing energy

outward citrus peel, peppermint, mint – dispersing outward flowing energy

Table 3 below lists various ingredients used in smoothies and their effect on energy flow direction.

Table 3 – Foods effect on energy flow

Energy flow	Ingredients
downward energy	Carrots, peeled ginger, sea salt
upward energy	Sprouts, asparagus, leeks
inward energy	vinegar
outward energy	Citrus peels, peppermint, spearmint, ginger peel

Using food color as a tool for energetic balancing

Food colors are used to help balance the smoothie in several ways. As described in preceding section scientific research has shown that different colors relate to different types of antioxidants found in the skin of fruit and vegetables. However, according to TCM different colors may also indicate an affinity to organs systems. This should only be taken as a general guideline as there are many exceptions to the rule. The core balanced smoothie combines colors related to various organ systems for example: tomatoes are red and related to the heart and blood vessels, chia seeds are black and related to the kidneys, ginger is yellow and is related to the digestive system. Table 4 below lists various ingredients used in smoothies and how their colors relate to the five organ systems.

Table 4 – How food colors relate to organ systems

Color	related organ system	Ingredients
White	Lungs and large intestine	Onions, garlic, radish, winter melon
Red	Cardiovascular system	Red peppers, tomatoes, dates, red chilies
Yellow/Brown	Digestive system	Ginger, yellow capsicum
Green	Liver and Gallbladder	Greens, Sprouts, cucumber
Black	Kidneys and Bladder	Black sesame and black chia seeds

Using food flavors as a tool for energetic balancing

Foods have complex flavors that often consists of two or three flavors. For example, a tomato is both sweet and sour. According to TCM food flavor(s) may indicate organ system(s) affected. This should only be taken as a general guideline as there are many exceptions to the rule. The core balanced smoothie recipe contains ingredients with various flavors that balance each other out. For example – berries and tomatoes are sweet and sour, pickled ginger is pungent, sweet and sour, Celtic sea salt and spinach are salty, apple cider vinegar (ACV) is sour and sweet, pawpaw and nigella seeds are bitter and pungent, some green leaves can be somewhat bitter (e.g. chard, rocket). Table 5 below lists various ingredients used in smoothies and how their flavors relate to the five organ systems.

Table 5 – How food flavors relate to organ systems

Flavor	related organ system	Ingredients
Pungent	Lungs and large intestine	Onions, garlic, leeks, radish, fresh ginger
Bitter	Cardiovascular system	Black nigella seeds, pawpaw seeds, coffee, rocket
Sweet	Digestive system	Tomatoes, some sweet fruit
Sour	Liver and Gallbladder	Lemons, tomatoes, vinegar, grapefruit
Salty	Kidneys and Bladder	Sea salt, Himalayan salt, seaweed

The examples in preceding sections demonstrate how foods can affect several organ systems. So to keep it simple the core balanced smoothie recipe includes a balanced synergistic combination of foods with diverse energetic properties, colors, and flavors in all these categories.

Seasonal balance

Traditional medicine maintains that each of the seasons has its own type of energy and accordingly a dominant organ system. Accordingly, different foods may be used in different seasons to support the energy type prevailing in that season. However, in modern times due to air-conditioning and heating systems the micro environment inside buildings and houses may be very different to the conditions outdoors both in temperature and humidity. So adjustments of your smoothies may depend more on your specific living, working and commuting environments than on the season. One way to keep things simple and stay in tune with nature is to try and eat locally grown, seasonal fruit and vegetables. That generally leads to a diet that is more compatible with seasonal and climatic conditions.

Individual balance

Traditional medicine maintains that diet has to be tailored holistically to the individual's constitution and condition. Some people have a weaker digestive system and are very sensitive to cold and windy conditions. They may prefer warm food and drinks. Others feel warm even in the winter, like to keep the windows open and prefer cold drinks and raw foods. Most people are somewhere in between. Iif you are a person who suffers from the cold in the winter, then you may consider reducing the quantities of cooling ingredients in your smoothies and increasing the quantities of warming and neutral ingredients listed above. In general, most green leaves, cucumbers and citrus fruit are rather cooling whereas ginger, cinnamon, pepper, turmeric, vinegar are warming or very warming. The smoothie should not taste too spicy. Smoothies are part of a daily diet that includes other foods with various energetic properties. It is the overall effect that matters.

SMOOTHIES FOR DIFFERENT DIETS & NEEDS

In a nutshell

The ideal diet is a widely debated subject beyond the scope of this book. I tend to go with the view that the diet needs to be personalized and tailored to suit a range of variables such as body type, constitution, life style, activity level, age, health status, climate and season to name a few.

We need to distinguish between omnivores, vegetarians, vegans and other special diets. Omnivore, vegetarian and vegan diets all have their strengths and weaknesses that are well beyond the scope of this book but their unique characteristics should be taken into consideration when designing your individualized smoothie.

Caution:

If you are suffering from any type of health condition, you may need to follow specific dietary guidelines. Accordingly, your smoothie also needs to take these guidelines into account. As stated in the disclaimer, this book is not a medical or nutritional guide for treating specific health conditions and therefore it is strongly advised that you seek the guidance of your doctor or health practitioner.

Smoothies for Omnivores

Omnivores are defined as people who eat a variety of foods of plant and animal sources. Omnivores are not restricted in their food sources and therefore have an easier time when shopping, preparing food and dining out and are less prone to develop various nutritional deficiencies than some vegans. On the downside food sourced from the animal kingdom tends to have a higher level of toxins because animals are higher up on the food chain than plants. Even organic meat, eggs and dairy may contain toxins due to contamination of the environment. Fish may contain mercury and radioactive isotopes. Even organically grown animals may accumulate toxins in their tissues due to incomplete detoxification of environmental and endogenous toxins. Therefore, when making smoothies, omnivores may benefit from having more emphasis on detoxification and prepare the detox smoothies more often. These are described in the following chapter "Making the Balanced Smoothies".

Smoothies for vegans

Vegans are defined as people who do not use animal products in their diet. A vegan diet has its advantages and disadvantages. On the upside consuming only plant based foods may help reduce exposure to some toxins that are more prevalent in animal based food.
On the downside strict vegan diets may increase the risk of developing a range of serious nutritional deficiencies that may build up over time. The symptoms may initially be subtle, diffuse and difficult to diagnose. The most common nutritional deficiencies that

may occur in some (but not all) vegans are deficiencies in vitamin B12, vitamin D3, heme-iron, DHA type omega-3 fatty acid, creatine, carnosine, taurine and sulfur. People have diverse genetic backgrounds and non-genetic (epigenetic) factors that are involved in switching genes on and off. This may partially explain why some people thrive on vegan diets where as others become unwell.

Vegans can prevent nutritional deficiencies by taking supplements and by using correct food combinations to consume an overall "complete" protein (e.g. rice and beans). If that doesn't work, they may consider adding a scoop of "complete" full spectrum protein vegan protein powder to their smoothies. The good brands usually have a mix of several vegan protein concentrates such as chia seed protein, hemp seed protein, pea protein and potato protein.

Vegans who consume a lot of legumes and grains may be getting too much omega-6 fatty acids and not enough omega-3 fatty acids. They may benefit by adding chia seeds and flaxseeds to their smoothies as these seeds are rich in omega-3 fatty acids vs omega-6 fatty acids.

Raw food vegans who consume only fruit, vegetables, seaweed, nuts and seeds are especially prone to protein deficiency. spirulina and chlorella are the best concentrated source of "complete" vegan protein containing about 57 percent complete protein in dry weight. However, spirulina and chlorella are rather expensive and some people are not big fans of the taste. Some seeds and nuts such as chia seeds, pumpkin seeds and pistachios also provide "complete" protein. However, a raw vegan would need to consume a cupful of seeds and nuts daily to get enough protein. Nuts and seeds are hard to digest and this would put a huge load on the digestive system and leave little energy for detoxification. Raw vegans may consider adding a scoop of "complete" full spectrum vegan protein powder to their smoothies to boost their protein intake without taxing the digestive system.

Remember – perfectionism may lead to ill health.

Smoothies for vegetarians

Vegetarians are nutritionally somewhere between omnivores and vegans. Vegetarians avoid fish and meat but may consume dairy products and eggs. Non-organic dairy and eggs may contain residues of antibiotics, hormones, pesticides, insecticides and GMO. Organic dairy produce and eggs probably contain much smaller levels of toxins. Therefore, when making their smoothies, vegetarians may benefit by putting some emphasis on detox but if their protein intake is low they may also consider boosting their smoothies with protein powder concentrate.

Smoothies for the Paleo diet

The Paleo diet is a special type of omnivore diet that aims to resemble the diet that the ancient people ate for millions of years before the agricultural era. It includes fruit, vegetables, meat, seafood, nuts and seeds. Some versions also include healthy fats. It does not include processed food and sugars, grains, legumes starches and dairy. The core balanced smoothie is for most part compatible with the Paleo diet. If your version of the Paleo diet excludes olive oil, you can use more avocados. If it excludes vinegar, use more lemon and lime juice.

Smoothies for sports

Athletes and people who engage in sports activities on a regular basis need to modify their dietary intake to take into account greater nutritional requirements and for detoxification of byproducts of sports activities. Dietary modifications depend on the frequency, intensity, duration and type of activity but in general there are several aspects that athletes and sports people need to address:

- **Increased energy expenditure**
- **Increased tissue wear and tear**
- **Increased muscle and bone tissue building**
- **Increased loss of electrolytes via sweating**
- **Increased formation of lactic acid in the muscles**

The body is able to generate energy from carbohydrates, fats and even proteins. The fuel with the quickest absorption and availability are simple sugars – glucose in particular. However, simple sugars are a very short term solution as excess is removed rapidly by the body, causing spikes in sugar and insulin levels in the blood. Complex carbohydrates are slower to break down and metabolize and generally have a lower GI (Glycemic index) factor and that helps regulate sugar and insulin levels in the blood while providing steady energy. Fats are slowest to digest and provide a good long term steady supply of energy. The best dietary fat for energy is coconut oil as it is very stable, doesn't go rancid easily and rich in MCTs (medium chain triglycerides) that provide a slow and sustained energy release while also boosting metabolism and fat loss. The core balanced smoothie recipe includes small amounts of sugars from berries and other fruit and small amounts of complex carbohydrates from fruit and vegetables. It also includes fats from seeds, avocado, olive oil and coconut oil (if room temperature is above 25 degrees Celsius and allows using coconut oil in the smoothie).

To repair tissue wear and tear and build muscle tissue, athletes and people engaged in sports, need more "complete" protein. The core balanced smoothie recipe is not intended to provide substantial amounts of protein. It includes small amounts of "complete" vegan protein from chia seeds, spirulina and chlorella. In order to boost the smoothie to provide substantial amounts of "complete" protein you can add a scoop of whey protein concentrate powder or a scoop of "full spectrum" vegan protein concentrate powder.

Athletes and sportspeople who train hard tend to sweat a lot especially when training outside in warm weather. This results in substantial loss of electrolytes that must be replenished promptly. The balanced smoothie naturally contains good amounts of electrolytes and by using coconut water (instead of water) and adding slightly more sea salt you can boost the smoothie's electrolytes levels further. This will provide a more natural, hydrating and alkalizing drink than most commercially available sports drinks, without artificial sweeteners, preservatives, colors, caffeine and commercial sugars. Sugar and caffeine may acidify, overstimulate and cause spikes in blood sugar level followed by spikes in insulin level. Caffeine may also have a diuretic effect leading to dehydration and thus defeating the purpose.

Lactic acid functions as a temporary fuel source for muscles during intense physical activity when normal glucose metabolism fails to provide enough energy. Presence of lactic acid in the muscles may cause a burning sensation. By improving glucose metabolism in the body the need for lactic acid is reduced. Fatty acids assist in glucose metabolism, B vitamins assist in glucose transfer and magnesium helps the body deliver energy to muscle cells. Seeds are rich in fatty acids and magnesium, green leafy vegetables are rich in magnesium and in B6 and Folate. Vitamin B12 is not present in most vegan food sources but whey protein concentrate does provide moderate amounts of B12. The core balanced smoothie recipe boosted with a scoop of whey protein concentrate provides magnesium, fatty acids and vitamins B6, Folate and B12 that will help improve energy metabolism and reduce the need for lactic acid.

HOW TO MAKE THE BALANCED SMOOTHIES

General procedure

1. Choose a recipe

2. Place all ingredients and tools on kitchen counter-top. Use the ingredient substitutions table below to substitute missing ingredients.

3. If using goji berries soak in water for 1 hour before using.

4. Wash and drain all fruit and vegetables

5. Cut fruit and vegetables to small slices to allow easy blending

6. Pour special liquids (e.g. coconut water, aloe Vera juice) into blender jug following the recipe. If no special liquids are required go to the next step.

7. Top up with water until reaching the correct liquid level for the intended number of serves (e.g. for 2 serves the total is between 1 cup and $1^1/_4$ cups). Liquid level should always be above the blender's blades to enable effective blending and prevent damage to the blender.

8. Add sliced fruit and vegetables.

9. Where peeled lemon or lime is specified you may opt for squeezing the lemon or lime and using only the juice. Blending the peeled lemon or lime adds more fiber and slight bitter flavor. Some like it and some don't.

10. Put the correct amounts of seeds into seed/coffee grinder and grind using several short pulses (to prevent overheating).

11. Scoop out ground seeds using a plastic spoon and add to blender jug Secure blender jug and jug cover

12. If your blender has a smoothie mode button use it. If not, blend for 30 to 60 seconds using the most suitable mode.

13. If the blender seems to be "struggling" stop it immediately, add a bit more water and try again. If slices of fruit or vegetables are still visible use the "Pulse" mode briefly several times to release any stuck slices and go back to normal mode.

14. Pour smoothie from blender jug into the mugs/bowls

15. Add olive oil as specified in the recipe and stir well with a spoon

16. Enjoy the smoothie **immediately** to minimize oxidation

Warnings:

1. To prevent damage or motor burnout stop the blender if it seems "stuck" or the sound is not right. Add water and try again. Use pulse mode a few time and try again. This may be the result of large vegetable or fruit slices stuck under the blades or an inadequate quantity of liquids.

2. To prevent damage or motor burnout stop the seed grinder if it seems "stuck" or the sound is not right. After a few seconds of grinding, some of the oil content of the seeds is

expelled and that may cause the ground seeds to stick together at the bottom of the grinder.

Ingredient substitutions

Table 6 below will help you find substitutes for ingredients you are missing, or for ingredients you just don't like, in a way that will not have a great impact on the overall balance nutritionally and energetically. Substitute a missing ingredient with an ingredient from the same row in the table. Try to use similar weight/volume as in the recipe.

Table 6 – Ingredient substitutions

Category	Ingredients	wt./volume (serves 2)
Green leafy vegetables	kale, spinach, sweet potato leaves, silver-beet, chard	2 cups total
Green garnish vegetables	parsley, cilantro, basil	¼ cup total
Other green vegetables	cucumber, green capsicum, celery	140 gm total
Other red/ orange vegetables	Red tomato, orange tomato, red capsicum, yellow capsicum	270 gm total
Sprouts	alfalfa, broccoli, radish, onion, garlic, Chinese cabbage	40 gm
Berries	goji berries, blueberries, raspberries, strawberries, cranberries, blackberries, boysenberries	1 Tbsp (dry), 2 Tbsp (fresh)
Low sugar citrus fruit	Lemon, lime	½ lemon or 1 lime

Other low sugar Fruit	Avocado, kiwi, granny smith apples	50 gm
Sweet fruit (use sparingly)	Papaya, guava, pineapple, custard apple, apples, pears, winter pears, grapes	25 gm
Cooling fruit (use sparingly)	Watermelon, all melons	25 gm
Omega-3 rich Seeds	Chia seeds, flax seeds,	1 tsp total
Other seeds	black cumin (nigella sativa), pumpkin, sunflower, pawpaw	1 tsp total
Oils	olive oil, coconut oil, (avocado fruit NOT oil)	4 Tbsp oil, ½ avocado
Salt	Celtic sea salt, Himalayan salt	A dash
Condiments	Apple cider vinegar (ACV)	1 tsp
Pickles	Pickled ginger, pickled beetroot (pickled with ACV)	1 Tbsp each
Seaweed	Nori seaweed	⅓ sheet
Liquids and juices	Water, coconut water, aloe Vera juice, beetroot juice, pomegranate juice, carrot juice, water kefir, kombucha	1 – 1/4 cup
Super-food supplements	spirulina, chlorella, wheatgrass, Barley green powders	2 tsp total
Protein supplements	Whey protein, "complete" vegan protein concentrates	Usually 1 scoop

BALANCED SMOOTHIE SYSTEM RECIPES

Intro

This section includes 21 balanced smoothie recipes. **The Core Balanced Smoothie** and **the Boosted Balanced Smoothie** are the ones I personally use most often. When I feel my body needs a bit of detox I use the **Core Detox Smoothie** or for extra detox I use the **Super Detox Smoothie**. When I suspect the environment or my lifestyle are creating a higher load of free radicals I use the **Core Antioxidant Smoothie** or for extra antioxidant support I use the **Super Antioxidant Smoothie. The sports smoothies** are designed as additional daily smoothies (not instead of the core smoothies). When I engage in sports activities I use the **Core Sports Smoothie** as an **additional** daily smoothie. For more demanding sports activities, I use the **Boosted Sports Smoothie** as an **additional** daily smoothie and for sports and outdoor activities that result in lots of sweating I use the **Sports Super Hydration smoothie** as an **additional** daily smoothie(s). **The Women's health support smoothie** and **Men's health support smoothie** put more emphasis on issues that are more common in women and men respectively, especially with age. **The spring, summer, autumn and winter smoothies** are designed **as additional daily** smoothies to help create better seasonal and energetic balance. There are three summer smoothies: **Light Cooling Summer Smoothie, Cooling Summer Smoothie and Super Cooling Green Tea Summer Smoothie** . As their names suggests each has a different level of cooling effect.

The black tea chai, cocoa and coffee based smoothies are very nice and designed as additional daily treats or energizers for lovers of cocoa, chai and coffee. And **the super creamy smoothie** is also a really nice additional daily treat. The following smoothies recipes are included:

1. Core Balanced Smoothie
2. Boosted Balanced Smoothie
3. Core Detox Smoothie
4. Super Detox Smoothie
5. Core Antioxidant Smoothie
6. Super Antioxidant Smoothie
7. Core Sports Smoothie
8. Boosted Sports Smoothie
9. Sports Super Hydration Smoothie
10. Women's Health Support Smoothie
11. Men's Health Support Smoothie
12. Balanced Spring Smoothie
13. Light Cooling Summer Smoothie
14. Cooling Summer Smoothie
15. Super Cooling Green Tea Summer Smoothie
16. Balanced Autumn Smoothie
17. Balanced Winter Smoothie
18. Sweet & Spicy Black Tea Smoothie
19. Energizing Sweet & Spicy Wake Up Coffee Smoothie
20. Super Thick Creamy Smoothie
21. Cocoa Delight Thick Creamy Smoothie

Core Balanced Smoothie

Ingredients (Serves 2)

- 1 cup water (or slightly more)
- 2 cups young leaves in total (spinach and/or silver beet and/or kale)
- ½ cup in total of parsley and/or cilantro leaves
- ½ cup sprouts (broccoli and/or alfalfa)
- 1 medium celery stalk with leaves
- 1 medium red capsicum
- 1 medium tomato
- 1 medium cucumber
- ½ peeled lemon
- 1 tsp shredded lemon rind (ONLY if using organic non-waxed lemon)
- 2 Tbs blueberries (fresh or frozen) OR 1 Tbs goji berries (dry)
- 1 Tbs pickled ginger (see pickling instructions)
- 2 Tbs pickled beetroot (see pickling instructions)
- 1 tsp flaxseeds
- 1 tsp chia seeds
- ½ tsp black nigella seeds
- ½ tsp pumpkin seeds
- ½ tsp black sesame seeds
- ½ tsp sunflower seeds
- 1/3 sheet of Nori seaweed

- 4 Tbs olive oil
- 1 dash of Celtic sea salt

Preparation

Follow the general smoothie preparation procedure described above. After serving the smoothie into mugs/bowls add 2 Tbs olive oil to each mug and stir well.

Write your notes here:

Boosted Balanced Smoothie

Ingredients (Serves 2)

- 1 cup water (or slightly more)
- 2 cups young leaves in total (spinach and/or silver beet and/or kale)
- ½ cup in total of parsley and/or cilantro leaves
- ½ cup sprouts (broccoli and/or alfalfa)
- 1 medium celery stalk with leaves
- 1 medium red capsicum
- 1 medium tomato
- 1 medium cucumber
- ½ peeled lemon
- 1 tsp shredded lemon rind (ONLY if using organic non-waxed lemon)
- 2 Tbs blueberries (fresh or frozen) OR 1 Tbs goji berries (dry)
- 1 Tbs pickled ginger (see pickling instructions)
- 2 Tbs pickled beetroot (see pickling instructions)
- 1 tsp flaxseeds
- 1 tsp chia seeds
- ½ tsp black nigella seeds
- ½ tsp pumpkin seeds
- ½ tsp black sesame seeds
- ½ tsp sunflower seeds
- 1/3 sheet of Nori seaweed

- 1 tsp spirulina powder

- 1 tsp chlorella powder

- 1 tsp wheatgrass powder

- 1 tsp barley green powder

- 2 Tbs olive oil

- 2 Tbs coconut oil

- 1 dash of Celtic sea salt

Preparation

Follow general smoothie preparation procedure described above. After serving the smoothie into mugs add oils to each mug and stir well. If room temperature is below 77°F (25°C), first liquefy the coconut oil in a saucepan on low heat, add 1 Tbs coconut oil to each mug and stir well. Drink immediately.

Write your notes here:

Core Detox Smoothie

Ingredients (Serves 2)

- 1 cup water (or slightly more)
- 1 cup cilantro leaves
- 1 cup parsley leaves
- ½ cup sprouts (broccoli and/or alfalfa)
- 1 medium celery stalk with leaves
- 1 medium red capsicum
- 1 medium tomato
- 1 medium cucumber
- ½ peeled lemon
- 1 tsp shredded lemon rind (ONLY if using organic non-waxed lemon)
- 1 Tbs goji berries (dry)
- 1 Tbs pickled ginger (see pickling instructions)
- 2 Tbs pickled beetroot (see pickling instructions)
- 1/3 sheet of Nori seaweed
- 4 Tbs olive oil
- 2 tsp chlorella
- ¼ tsp turmeric powder
- 1 dash black pepper powder
- 1 dash of Celtic sea salt

Preparation

Follow the general procedure described above. After serving the smoothie into mugs add 2 Tbs olive oil to each mug and stir well.

Write your notes here:

Super Detox Smoothie

Ingredients (Serves 2)

- ½ cup water (or slightly more)
- ¼ cup aloe Vera juice
- ¼ cup beetroot juice
- 1 cup cilantro leaves
- 1 cup parsley leaves
- ¼ cup rocket leaves
- ½ cup sprouts (broccoli and/or alfalfa)
- 1 medium celery stalk with leaves
- 1 medium red capsicum
- 1 medium tomato
- 1 medium cucumber
- ½ peeled lemon
- 1 tsp shredded lemon rind (ONLY if using organic non-waxed lemon)
- 1 Tbs goji berries (dry)
- 1 Tbs pickled ginger (see pickling instructions)
- 4 Tbs olive oil
- 1 Tbs chlorella
- 1 tsp spirulina powder
- 1 tsp wheatgrass powder
- 1 tsp barley green powder
- ½ tsp turmeric powder

- 1 dash black pepper powder

- 1 dash of Celtic sea salt

Preparation

Serve the smoothie then add 2 Tbs of olive oil to each of the mugs and stir well.

Write your notes here:

Core Antioxidant Smoothie

- Ingredients (Serves 2)
- ½ cup water (or slightly more)
- ¼ cup beetroot juice
- ¼ cup pomegranate juice
- 2 cups young leaves in total (spinach and/or silver beet and/or kale)
- ½ cup in total of parsley and/or cilantro leaves
- ½ cup sprouts (broccoli and/or alfalfa)
- 1 medium celery stalk with leaves
- 1 small red capsicum
- 1 small tomato
- 1 small cucumber
- 1 small peeled and seeded avocado
- ½ peeled lemon
- 1 tsp shredded lemon rind (ONLY if using organic non-waxed lemon)
- 4 Tbs blueberries (fresh or frozen)
- 2 Tbs goji berries (dry)
- 1 Tbs pickled ginger (see pickling instructions)
- ½ tsp flaxseeds
- ½ tsp chia seeds
- ½ tsp black nigella seeds
- ½ tsp black sesame seeds
- 1/3 sheet of Nori seaweed

- ¼ tsp turmeric powder

- 1 dash of black pepper

- 4 Tbs olive oil

- 1 dash of Celtic sea salt

Preparation

Follow the general smoothie preparation procedure described above. After serving the smoothie into mugs/bowls add 2 Tbs olive oil to each mug and stir well.

<u>**Write your notes here:**</u>

Super Antioxidant Smoothie

Ingredients (Serves 2)

- ½ cup strong COLD green tea (or slightly more)

- ¼ cup beetroot juice

- ¼ cup pomegranate juice

- 2 cups young leaves in total (spinach and/or silver beet and/or kale)

- ½ cup in total of parsley and/or cilantro leaves

- ½ cup sprouts (broccoli and/or alfalfa)

- 1 medium celery stalk with leaves

- 1 small red capsicum

- 1 small tomato

- 1 small cucumber

- 1 kiwi fruit

- ½ peeled lemon

- 1 tsp shredded lemon rind (ONLY if using organic non-waxed lemon)

- 4 Tbs blueberries (fresh or frozen)

- 2 Tbs goji berries (dry)

- 1 Tbs pickled ginger (see pickling instructions)

- ½ tsp flaxseeds

- ½ tsp chia seeds

- ½ tsp black nigella seeds

- ½ tsp black sesame seeds

- 1/3 sheet of Nori seaweed

- ½ tsp turmeric powder

- 1 dash of black pepper

- 4 Tbs olive oil

- 1 dash of Celtic sea salt

Preparation

1. Let tea cool down to room temperature BEFORE adding to other ingredients in the blender jug!!!

2. Follow the general smoothie preparation procedure described above.

3. After serving the smoothie into mugs/bowls add 2 Tbs olive oil to each mug and stir well.

Write your notes here:

Basic Sports Smoothie

Ingredients (Serves 2)

- 1 cup water (or slightly more)
- ¼ cup beetroot juice
- 2 cups young leaves in total (spinach and/or silver beet and/or kale)
- ½ cup in total of parsley and/or cilantro leaves
- ½ cup sprouts (broccoli and/or alfalfa)
- 1 medium celery stalk with leaves
- 1 small red capsicum
- 1 small tomato
- 1 small cucumber
- ½ peeled lemon
- 1 tsp shredded lemon rind (ONLY if using organic non-waxed lemon)
- 4 Tbs blueberries (fresh or frozen) OR 2 Tbs goji berries (dry)
- 1 Tbs pickled ginger (see pickling instructions)
- 4 Tbs olive oil
- 1 dash of Celtic sea salt
- 1 scoop whey protein concentrate or 1 scoop complete vegan protein concentrate

Preparation

1. Follow the general procedure described above.
2. After serving the smoothie into mugs add protein powder

concentrate

3. Add 2 Tbs of olive oil to each of the mugs and stir well

Write your notes here:

Boosted Sports Smoothie

Ingredients (Serves 2)

- 1 cup water (or slightly more)
- ½ cup beetroot juice
- 2 cups young leaves in total (spinach and/or silver beet and/or kale)
- ½ cup in total of parsley and/or cilantro leaves
- ½ cup sprouts (broccoli and/or alfalfa)
- 1 medium celery stalk with leaves
- 1 small red capsicum
- 1 small tomato
- 1 small cucumber
- ½ peeled lemon
- 1 tsp shredded lemon rind (ONLY if using organic non-waxed lemon)
- 4 Tbs blueberries (fresh or frozen) OR 2 Tbs goji berries (dry)
- 1 Tbs pickled ginger (see pickling instructions)
- 3 tsp chia seeds
- 1 tsp pumpkin seeds
- ½ tsp black nigella seeds
- 2 Tbs olive oil
- 2 Tbs coconut oil
- ½ tsp turmeric powder
- 1 dash of black pepper

- 1 dash of Celtic sea salt
- 1 scoop whey protein concentrate or 1 scoop complete vegan protein concentrate

Preparation

1. Follow the general procedure described above.
2. After serving the smoothie add oils to each mug and stir well.

Note:

If room temperature is below 77°F (25°C), first liquefy the coconut oil in a saucepan on low heat, add 1 Tbs to each mug and stir well.

<u>Write your notes here:</u>

Sports Super Hydration Smoothie

Ingredients (Serves 2)

- 1 cup coconut water (or slightly more)
- ¼ cup beetroot juice
- 2 cups young leaves in total (spinach and/or silver beet and/or kale)
- ½ cup in total of parsley and/or cilantro leaves
- ½ cup sprouts (broccoli and/or alfalfa)
- 1 medium celery stalk with leaves
- 1 small red capsicum
- 1 small tomato
- 1 large cucumber
- ½ peeled lemon
- 1 tsp shredded lemon rind (ONLY if using organic non-waxed lemon)
- 2 Tbs blueberries (fresh or frozen) OR 1 Tbs goji berries (dry)
- 1/3 sheet of Nori seaweed
- 1 Tbs pickled ginger (see pickling instructions)
- 4 Tbs olive oil
- 1 dash of Celtic sea salt

Preparation

1. Follow the general procedure described above.
2. After serving the smoothie into mugs add protein powder

3.   Add 2 Tbs of olive oil to each of the mugs and stir well.

<u>Write your notes here:</u>

Women's health support smoothie

Ingredients (Serves 2)

- ½ cup water (or slightly more)
- ½ cup cranberry juice (preferably organic with no added sugar, colors or preservatives)
- 2 cups young leaves in total (spinach and/or silver beet and/or kale)
- ½ cup in total of parsley and/or cilantro leaves
- ½ cup sprouts (broccoli and/or alfalfa)
- 1 medium celery stalk with leaves
- 1 small red capsicum
- 1 small tomato
- 1 small cucumber
- ¼ cup sliced fennel bulb (if available)
- ¼ cup sliced onion
- ½ peeled lemon
- 1 tsp shredded lemon rind (ONLY if using organic non-waxed lemon)
- 1 Tbs cranberries (fresh or frozen)
- 1 Tbs blueberries (fresh or frozen) OR 1 Tbs goji berries (dry)
- 1 Tbs pickled ginger (see pickling instructions)
- 2 Tbs pickled beetroot (see pickling instructions)
- 2 tsp flaxseeds
- 1 tsp psyllium seed husks
- ½ tsp black nigella seeds

- ½ tsp black sesame seeds
- 1/3 sheet of Nori seaweed
- ¼ tsp turmeric powder
- 1 dash of black pepper
- 4 Tbs olive oil
- 1 dash of Celtic sea salt

Preparation

Follow the general procedure described above. After serving add oils to each mug and stir well. If room temperature is below 77°F (25°C), first liquefy coconut oil in a saucepan on low heat, add 1 Tbs to each mug and stir well.

Write your notes here:

Men's Health Support Smoothie

Ingredients (Serves 2)

- ½ cup water (or slightly more)
- ½ cup tomato juice
- 2 cups young leaves in total (spinach and/or silver beet and/or kale)
- ½ cup in total of parsley and/or cilantro leaves
- ½ cup sprouts (broccoli and/or alfalfa)
- 1 medium celery stalk with leaves
- 1 small red capsicum
- 1 small cucumber
- ½ peeled lemon
- 1 tsp shredded lemon rind (ONLY if using organic non-waxed lemon)
- 2 Tbs blueberries (fresh or frozen) OR 1 Tbs goji berries (dry)
- 1 Tbs pickled ginger (see pickling instructions)
- 2 Tbs pickled beetroot (see pickling instructions)
- 2 tsp pumpkin seeds
- ½ tsp black nigella seeds
- ½ tsp black sesame seeds
- 1 tsp psyllium seed husks
- 1/3 sheet of Nori seaweed
- ¼ tsp turmeric powder
- 1 dash of black pepper

- 2 Tbs olive oil
- 2 Tbs coconut oil
- 1 dash of Celtic sea salt

Preparation

1. Follow the general procedure described above
2. After serving the smoothie into mugs add oils to each mug and stir well.
3. If room temperature is below 77°F (25°C), first liquefy the coconut oil in a saucepan on low heat, add 1 Tbs to each mug and stir well.

<u>Write your notes here:</u>

Balanced Spring Smoothie

Ingredients (Serves 2)

- 1 cup water (or slightly more)
- 2 cups young leaves in total (watercress and/or spinach and/or silver beet and/or kale)
- ½ cup sprouts (broccoli and/or alfalfa)
- ½ medium avocado
- ½ medium fennel bulb (if available)
- 1 or 2 peeled limes
- 1 tsp shredded lime rind (ONLY if using organic non-waxed lime)
- 2 Tbs blueberries (fresh or frozen) OR 1 Tbs goji berries (dry)
- 2 tsp chia seeds
- 1 tsp pumpkin seeds
- 4 Tbs olive oil
- 1 dash of Celtic sea salt

Preparation

Follow the general smoothie preparation procedure described above. After serving the smoothie into mugs/bowls add 2 Tbs olive oil to each mug and stir well.

Write your notes here:

Light Cooling Summer Smoothie

Ingredients (Serves 2)

- ¾ cup water (or slightly more)
- 2 cups young leaves in total (spinach and/or silver beet and/or kale)
- ½ cup in total of parsley and/or cilantro leaves
- ½ cup sprouts (broccoli and/or alfalfa)
- ½ cup melon
- ½ cup watermelon
- ½ peeled lemon
- 1 tsp shredded lemon rind (ONLY if using organic non-waxed lemon)
- 2 Tbs blueberries (fresh or frozen) OR 1 Tbs goji berries (dry)
- 2 tsp chia seeds
- 4 Tbs olive oil
- 1 dash of Celtic sea salt

Preparation

Follow the general smoothie preparation procedure described above. After serving the smoothie into mugs/bowls add 2 Tbs olive oil to each mug and stir well.

Write your notes here:

Cooling Summer Smoothie

Ingredients (Serves 2)

- ¾ cup water (or slightly more)
- 2 cups young leaves in total (spinach and/or silver beet and/or kale)
- ½ cup in total of parsley and/or cilantro leaves
- ½ cup sprouts (broccoli and/or alfalfa)
- ¼ cup mint leaves
- ½ cup melon
- ½ cup watermelon
- ½ peeled lemon
- 1 tsp shredded lemon rind (ONLY if using organic non-waxed lemon)
- 2 Tbs blueberries (fresh or frozen) OR 1 Tbs goji berries (dry)
- 2 tsp chia seeds
- 4 Tbs olive oil
- 1 dash of Celtic sea salt

Preparation

Follow the general smoothie preparation procedure described above. After serving the smoothie into mugs/bowls add 2 Tbs olive oil to each mug and stir well.

Write your notes here:

Super Cooling Summer Green Tea Smoothie

Ingredients (Serves 2)

- ¾ cup COLD green tea (or slightly more)
- 2 cups young leaves in total (spinach and/or silver beet and/or kale)
- ½ cup in total of parsley and/or cilantro leaves
- ¼ cup mint leaves
- ½ cup sprouts (broccoli and/or alfalfa)
- ½ cup melon
- ½ cup watermelon
- ½ peeled lemon
- 1 tsp shredded lemon rind (ONLY if using organic non-waxed lemon)
- 2 Tbs blueberries (fresh or frozen) OR 1 Tbs goji berries (dry)
- 2 tsp chia seeds
- 4 Tbs olive oil
- 1 dash of Celtic sea salt

Preparation

1. Let tea cool down to room temperature **BEFORE** adding to other ingredients in the blender jug!!!
2. Follow the general smoothie preparation procedure described above.
3. After serving the smoothie into mugs/bowls add 2 Tbs olive oil to each mug and stir well.

Write your notes here:

Balanced Autumn Smoothie

Ingredients (Serves 2)

- 1 cup water (or slightly more)
- 2 cups young leaves in total (spinach and/or silver beet and/or kale)
- ½ cup in total of parsley and/or cilantro leaves
- ¼ cup in total of basil and/or coriander leaves
- ½ medium celery stalk with leaves
- 1 medium red capsicum
- 1 medium tomato
- ¼ peeled lemon
- 1 tsp shredded lemon rind (ONLY if using organic non-waxed lemon)
- 2 Tbs cranberries (fresh or frozen)
- 1 Tbs pickled ginger (see pickling instructions)
- 2 Tbs pickled beetroot (see pickling instructions)
- 1 tsp flaxseeds
- 1 tsp chia seeds
- ½ tsp black nigella seeds
- ½ tsp pumpkin seeds
- 1 tsp apple cider vinegar (ACV)
- ¼ tsp turmeric powder
- 1 dash black pepper powder
- 4 Tbs olive oil
- 1 dash of Celtic sea salt

Preparation

Follow the general smoothie preparation procedure described above. After serving the smoothie into mugs/bowls add 2 Tbs olive oil to each mug and stir well.

Write your notes here:

Balanced Winter Smoothie

Ingredients (Serves 2)

- 1 cup water (or slightly more)
- 2 cups young leaves in total (spinach and/or silver beet and/or kale)
- ½ cup in total of parsley and/or cilantro leaves
- ¼ cup in total of basil and/or coriander leaves
- ½ medium celery stalk with leaves
- 1 medium red capsicum
- 1 medium tomato
- ¼ peeled lemon
- 1 tsp shredded lemon rind (ONLY if using organic non-waxed lemon)
- 2 Tbs cranberries (fresh or frozen)
- 1 Tbs pickled ginger (see pickling instructions)
- 2 Tbs pickled beetroot (see pickling instructions)
- 1 tsp black sesame seeds
- 1 tsp flaxseeds
- 1 tsp chia seeds
- ½ tsp black nigella seeds
- 1 tsp apple cider vinegar (ACV)
- ¼ tsp cinnamon powder
- ¼ tsp turmeric powder
- 1 dash black pepper powder
- 4 Tbs olive oil

- 1 dash of Celtic sea salt

Preparation

Follow the general smoothie preparation procedure described above. After serving the smoothie into mugs/bowls add 2 Tbs olive oil to each mug and stir well.

<u>Write your notes here:</u>

Sweet and Spicy Black Tea Chai Smoothie

Ingredients (Serves 2)

- ½ cup COLD strong black tea (or slightly more)
- ½ cup unsweetened almond milk
- ½ cup unsweetened coconut milk
- 1 medium size winter pear
- 2 pitted meddlesome dates
- 2 Tbs blueberries (fresh or frozen)
- 1 Tbs goji berries (dry)
- 1 tsp black sesame seeds
- 1 tsp flaxseeds
- 1 tsp chia seeds
- ½ tsp black nigella seeds
- 1 tsp shredded tangerine or orange rind (ONLY if using organic non-waxed fruit)
- ¼ tsp cinnamon powder
- ½ tsp ginger powder
- ½ tsp cardamom powder
- ¼ tsp fennel powder or anise powder
- 1 dash clove powder
- 1 dash black pepper powder
- a few drops of stevia extract to taste (optional)

Preparation

1. Bring water to a boil. Add spices (cinnamon, cardamom,

ginger, black pepper) and simmer for 5 minutes.

2. Add 2 bags of black tea. Let simmer for another 2 minutes. Take out teabags.

3. Add unsweetened coconut milk to tea and stir well

4. Add unsweetened almond milk to tea and stir well

5. Let liquids **COOL DOWN** to room temperature **BEFORE** adding to other ingredients in the blender jug!!!

6. Follow the general smoothie preparation procedure described above.

Notes:

1. This smoothie has a higher caloric value than most smoothies in this book because it includes more fruit, almond milk and coconut milk.

2. An easier, although slightly costlier way to prepare the black chai smoothie is to use 2 teabags of your favorite readymade black chai tea instead of putting all the ingredients together yourself (i.e. mixing the spices and the black tea).

Write your notes here:

Energizing Sweet & Spicy Wake Up Coffee Smoothie

Ingredients (Serves 2)

- 1 cup COLD strong black coffee (or slightly more)
- ½ cup unsweetened almond milk
- ½ medium banana
- 2 pitted medjool dates
- 3 Tbs blueberries (fresh or frozen)
- 1 tsp black sesame seeds
- 1 tsp flaxseeds
- 1 tsp chia seeds
- ½ tsp black nigella seeds
- ¼ tsp ginger powder
- ½ tsp cardamom powder
- a few drops of stevia extract to taste (optional)

Preparation:

1. Make black coffee, add spices and stir well
2. Add unsweetened almond milk to coffee and stir well
3. Let liquids **COOL DOWN** to room temperature **BEFORE** adding to other ingredients in the blender jug!!!
4. Follow the general smoothie preparation procedure described above.

Notes:

1.   This smoothie has a higher caloric value than most smoothies in this book because it includes more fruit and almond milk.

2.   **Not suitable just before bedtime.**

<u>Write your notes here:</u>

Super Thick Creamy Smoothie

Ingredients (Serves 2)

- ½ cup unsweetened almond milk (or slightly more)
- ½ cup coconut milk
- 2 cups young leaves in total (spinach and/or silver beet and/or kale)
- ½ cup in total of parsley and/or cilantro leaves
- ½ cup sprouts (broccoli and/or alfalfa)
- 1 medium celery stalk with leaves
- 1 medium peeled and pitted avocado
- ½ cup papaya / pawpaw
- ½ peeled lemon
- 1 tsp shredded lemon rind (ONLY if using organic non-waxed lemon)
- 2 Tbs blueberries (fresh or frozen) OR 1 Tbs goji berries (dry)
- 1 Tbs pickled ginger (see pickling instructions)
- 2 Tbs pickled beetroot (see pickling instructions)
- 1 tsp flaxseeds
- 1 tsp chia seeds
- ½ tsp black nigella seeds
- ½ tsp pumpkin seeds
- ½ tsp black sesame seeds
- ½ tsp sunflower seeds
- 1/3 sheet of Nori seaweed

- 2 Tbs olive oil
- 1 dash of Celtic sea salt

Preparation

Follow the general smoothie preparation procedure described above.

Note:

This smoothie has a higher caloric value than most smoothies as it includes pawpaw, coconut milk and almond milk.

<u>Write your notes here:</u>

Cocoa Delight Thick Creamy Smoothie

Ingredients (Serves 2)

- ½ cup unsweetened almond milk (or slightly more)
- ½ cup unsweetened coconut milk
- ½ medium banana
- ½ medium avocado
- 2 pitted medjool dates
- 3 Tbs blueberries (fresh or frozen)
- 1 tsp black sesame seeds
- 1 tsp flaxseeds
- 1 tsp chia seeds
- ½ tsp black nigella seeds
- ¼ tsp ginger powder
- ¼ tsp cinnamon powder
- 4 Tbs raw unsweetened cocoa powder
- a few drops of stevia extract to taste (optional)

Preparation:

1. Mix cocoa powder, spices with liquids and add to blender jug.
2. Blend for a few seconds until the mixture is uniform
3. Follow general procedure for the seeds and other ingredients
4. Blend well until extra smooth.

Note:

This smoothie has a higher caloric value than most smoothies in this book because it includes more fruit and almond milk.

<u>Write your notes here:</u>

ADDING THICKNESS & TEXTURE

Some ingredients can make your smoothies thicker, creamier or add texture. The table below will help you choose texturizing ingredients.

Table 7 - Adding thickness to smoothies

Note: Quantities shown for 1 serve.			
Ingredient	**Effect on smoothie**	**Quantity**	**comments**
Chia seeds	thicker, heavier	1 tsp	See comment # 1
Flax-seeds	thicker, heavier	1 tsp	See comment # 1
psyllium husks	thicker	1 tsp	See comment # 2
Coconut flour	thicker, heavier	2 tsp	See comment # 3
Avocado	thicker, creamy	½ -1 avocado	See comment # 4
Mango	thicker, creamier, sweeter	½ small mango	
Banana	thicker, heavier, creamier, sweeter	½ -1 banana	
Guava	thicker, heavier, creamier, sweeter	1 guava	
Coconut milk	thicker, creamier, heavier, sweeter	½ cup	
Almond milk	creamier, sweeter	1 - ½ cup	
Coconut oil	creamier, oily	1 Tbs	See comment # 5
Olive oil	creamier, oily	1 Tbs	See comment # 6
Orange peel	thicker, heavier, tangy	2 tsp ground rind	See comment # 7
Lemon peel	thicker, heavier, tangy	2 tsp ground rind	See comment # 7

Comments:

#1. Grind seeds in grinder. A gel forms when seeds come in contact with water. This makes cleaning some blenders time consuming. IF your blender is difficult to clean – mix with ¼ cup of water until ground seeds absorb some water and swell. Add to prepared smoothie in cup(s) not to jug. Stir well with a spoon.

#2. Mix with 1 cup of water until husks absorb water and swell before adding to other ingredients. A gel forms when husks come in contact with water. This makes cleaning some blenders time consuming. IF your blender is difficult to clean DO NOT add to blender jug with other ingredient. Add to smoothie after serving and stir with a spoon.

#3. Add liquids and stir a few times. After coconut flour has swollen add to liquids in blender.

#4. Avocado gives a lovely smooth creamy texture yet does not make the smoothie heavy. Can be used with both sweet and savory smoothies.

#5. Use only above room temperature of 24 Celsius (76 Fahrenheit). Coconut oil liquefies above this temperature and solidifies below it. Add to prepared smoothie in cup(s). Stir well with a spoon. DO NOT add to blender jug with other ingredient as this makes cleaning the blender time consuming.

#6. Add to prepared smoothie in cup(s). Stir well with a spoon. DO NOT add to blender jug with other ingredient as this makes cleaning the blender time consuming.

#7. Use ONLY organic citrus peel that have not been coated with wax. Non-organic peels may be covered with chemicals. Some organic citrus fruit are covered with wax to protect the fruit in transit and storage. DO NOT used the peels if they are waxed. To test for presence of wax place the peel in a bowl and pour boiling water over it. Wax will melt and stick to the bottom when water cools.

MAKING PICKLED VEGETABLES FOR SMOOTHIES

Making pickled ginger

Pickled ginger is an excellent condiment and a very important ingredient in the balanced smoothie recipe. It requires a bit of preparation but you only need to prepare a batch once every few months.

Pickled ginger has a warm energetic property that balances the cooling effect of green leafy vegetables, cucumbers, cabbage and other ingredients. Pickled ginger has four flavors: pungent, sweet, sour and salty that further enhance and balance the balanced smoothie flavor. Overall the combination of energetic properties and flavors greatly enhances digestion and absorption of all other ingredients. The following recipe is simple, quick and easy to make. It uses only three ingredients:

Ingredients:

- **1 lb. (453 gram) fresh ginger** – Use fresh, smooth skinned, large ginger roots. They are easier to clean, peel and slice. Stay away from old shriveled, rough ginger roots.
- **2 cups Apple cider vinegar (ACV)** – try to get organic, unfiltered with the "mother".
- **1 Tbs sea salt (or Himalayan salt)**

Preparation:

1. Clean and sterilize a 1 quart (almost 1 liter) glass jar.
2. Scrub the ginger roots with a brush and wash well.
3. Remove the skins using a vegetable peeler. Inspect to make sure the skins have been removed completely. Wash again to get rid of any remaining bits.
4. Slice the peeled ginger as thinly as you can (preferably paper thin) using a mandolin or grater.
5. Pour the ACV into the jar and add the salt. Stir well to dissolve the salt.
6. Add the sliced ginger and cover with the lid
7. Refrigerate the jar. It will be ready to use in 7 days and will keep in the fridge for several months.

Notes:

1. Many pickled ginger recipes use rice vinegar. I use ACV because of its superior health benefits. It is also more suitable for people who avoid all grains.
2. You can keep the ginger skins in a container in the freezer and use them for making ginger tea by boiling the skins and other ingredients for 5 -10 minutes and then straining into a cup. Waste not want not!

Cautions:

1. When slicing the ginger pay close attention and be careful not to slice your fingers in the process!

2. Make sure you let the ginger soak in the vinegar for 7 days before using it. Provided the slices are thin enough the concentrated vinegar will get rid of nasties that have managed to cling to the ginger.

Write your notes here:

Making pickled beetroot

Pickled beetroot is an excellent condiment and a recommended ingredient for the balanced smoothie recipe. It requires a bit of preparation but you only need to prepare a batch once every couple of weeks.

Pickled beetroot has three flavors: sweet, sour and salty that further enhance and balance the balanced smoothie flavor. Beetroot has excellent nutritional qualities as it is very high on antioxidants, and may help prevent cancer and cardiovascular disease. It may also enhance sports performance.

The following recipe is simple, quick and easy and to make. It uses only three ingredients:

Ingredients:

- **4 large beetroots** – Use fresh large beetroots.
- **2 cups Apple cider vinegar (ACV)**
- **1 Tbs sea salt (or Himalayan salt)**
- **1 bay leaf**
- **1 garlic clove**
- **2 whole cloves**

Preparation:

1. Clean and sterilize a 1 quart (almost 1 liter) glass jar.

2. Scrub the beetroots with a brush and wash well.

3. Put beetroots in a pot. Cover with water. Bring to a boil. Simmer for 5-10 minutes

4. Let cool. Remove water. Take beetroots out.

5. Peel skins and blemishes off using a vegetable peeler. Make sure the skins have been removed completely. Wash again to get rid of any remaining bits.

6. Slice beetroots thinly using a mandolin or grater.

7. Pour the ACV into the jar and add the salt. Stir well to dissolve the salt.

8. Add the sliced beetroot and cover with the lid

9. Refrigerate the jar. It will be ready to use in 7 days and will keep in the fridge for a few weeks.

Note:

Many pickled beetroot recipes use white vinegar. I use ACV because of its superior health benefits. It is also more suitable for people who avoid all grains. Try to get organic, unfiltered with the mother.

Cautions:

1. When slicing the beetroot pay close attention and be careful not to slice your fingers in the process!

2. Let the beetroot soak in the vinegar for 7 days **BEFORE** using it.

Write your notes here:

SMOOTHIE MAKING EQUIPMENT & TOOLS

Blenders

Best and worst blenders for smoothies

Some blenders are not suitable for making smoothies. Their motors may not be strong enough, their blades may be of poor quality, they may be difficult to clean or their design may not be suitable. If the motor is not strong enough it may not outlast the warranty. Cheap blades will wear out quickly and the smoothies will become grainy and not smooth at all. If the blades are not removable, cleaning will be difficult and vegetables fibers will get stuck under the blades.

A good blender has to be powerful enough (at least 850 watt), have tough hardened stainless steel removable blades that are easy to clean and a warranty for at least 2 or 3 years.

Some blenders have a smoothie mode button. This comes in handy because all you have to do is press the button once and the blender selects suitable time and sequence of varying speeds and pulses to loosen up vegetables and fruit that get stuck above the blades. The end result is a smoothie with a nice smooth texture indicating that all ingredients have been pulverized into small particles that ensure optimal digestion and absorption of nutrients.

Criteria for blender selection

- **Motor power**
- **Jug size**
- **Jug Material**
- **Overall blender size**
- **Configuration and design**
- **Convenience of disassembling and cleaning**

Motor power

Generally, you should be looking for a blender that is at least 850 watts although a smaller motor with very high quality blades may perform better than a larger motor with dull blades.

Jug size

Small jugs are more suitable for single serves and large jug sizes are more suitable for family size smoothies. Making a smoothie in blender with a large jug requires more liquids for the same quantity of ingredients. Often the end result will be 1.5 or even 2 serves even if you only want to make a single serve. So if you usually make single serves go for a blender with a small jug.

Jug material

Another consideration is the material the jug is made of. Some are made of glass but in most smaller models designed for single serves the jug is made of some type of food grade hardened plastic.

Blender types

Blending quality translates to higher nutrient availability and better nutritional outcomes so for those serious about making smoothies blender quality is important. There are several basic blender designs and each has advantages and disadvantages. However, some may not be suitable for making the balanced smoothie and some may not be suitable for other applications. Here are the main blender types:

Cheap hand held blenders

Hand held blenders also called stick blender or immersion blender are thin long hand held devices. Most have a relatively small motor (150 -200 W) and a relatively small blade configuration. They are useful for blending soups in the cooking pan (after the ingredients have already been cooked) and various other soft ingredients, thin drinks and thin smoothies. However, they are **NOT SUITABLE** for making the balanced smoothie and green smoothies in general because their motors are simply not strong enough and blade configuration too small to handle green leafy vegetable and other tough ingredients.

Cheap hand held blenders with attachments

These usually have more powerful motors (200 -500 W) than the basic cheap hand held blender. They usually come with several handy attachments including a measuring beaker that doubles as a blender jug, an attachment for chopping and one for whisking. They are useful for food chopping and whisking and for blending soups in the cooking pan (after the ingredients have already been cooked) and various soft ingredients, thin drinks and thin smoothies. However, they are **NOT SUITABLE** for making the balanced smoothie and green smoothies in general because their motors are simply not strong enough and blade configuration too small to handle green leafy vegetable and other tough ingredients.

Counter-top blenders

This type of blender includes a wide variety of sub-categories, designs and a wide range of price tags. In general counter top blenders are the most suitable for making the balanced smoothie because they have stronger motors and sturdier designs. Motor power ranges from 500 watts to 2000 watts. Generally, you should be looking for a blender that is at least 850 watts although a smaller motor with very high quality blades may perform better than a larger motor with dull blades. With traditional designs you pour the smoothie out of the jug into a cup(s). Some newer designs allow drinking the smoothie directly out of the jug. They often come with several jugs of different sizes. These designs are smaller, light weight and suitable for making a single serve and for busy people on the go that still want to maintain their health by consuming the balanced smoothie recipe daily.

Testing your blender

If you already have a blender test it a few times to see how well it works for making smoothies. If the blender has a dedicated smoothie setting, try it first. If the smoothies seem too chunky or grainy you may need to sharpen or replace the blades. With cheap blenders it may not be worth it. Even if you are on a limited budget then getting a cheap new counter-top blender may work out better than replacing or sharpening the blades. The problem with cheap blades is that often the coating wears off very quickly. In that case sharpening the blades may be counterproductive.

After testing your blender, try making the same smoothie with a better blender, perhaps go to a friend or relative who has a good blender and make the core balanced smoothie recipe together. If the result is smoother and more uniform, then you may consider getting a better blender simply because blending quality translates to higher nutrient availability and better nutritional outcomes.

Seed grinders and coffee bean grinders

Seed grinders are essential for grinding chia, black nigella and flax seeds. I use them to grind all seeds but some seeds like pumpkin seeds and sunflower seeds may be soaked overnight and then processed in the blender provided you have a good quality blender with effective blades. It doesn't work for chia and flax seeds because they absorb substantial amounts of water and form a thick gel. Traditional "manual" grinders allow grinding seeds slowly without a significant rise in temperature. This helps prevent the sensitive oil content (e.g. in flaxseed or chia seed) from being damaged by heat. The oil content in seeds makes most traditional manual coffee bean grinders ("hand" grinders) difficult to clean and therefore not suitable for grinding seeds. If you cannot find a specially designed "manual" seed grinder that is easy to clean then you may have to compromise and get an electric coffee grinder. Most are easy to clean and reasonably priced. Try to get one that has a stainless steel chamber. It is recommended that you do the grinding in short pulses. Press and hold for a second or two and then release. Repeat the process until the seeds are ground properly. This will prevent the grinder from overheating and extend the life of the motor. Use a wooden or plastic spoon to scoop the grind out of the grinder. Don't use a metal spoon as it may damage the blade or scratch the grinder.

Lemon zesters / micro-plane graters

The lemon zester and micro-plane grater are two common inexpensive kitchen tools used to obtain the zest from the top part of the rind of citrus fruit. For the balanced smoothie recipe, you may consider getting 1-2 teaspoons of zest from the lemon or lime before you cut and squeeze the juice out. The best are the ones that produce fine particles.

Citrus squeezer/juicer

The citrus squeezer is common inexpensive kitchen tool used to extract juice from citrus fruit by separating the juice from the pulp. They come in various sizes and for lemons and limes you only need a small simple squeezer made of plastic or glass.

ORGANIC, NON-ORGANIC AND GMO

Background

Until world war II most farm produce was organically grown and produced without the use of artificial fertilizers, herbicides, pesticides and fungicides. Unfortunately, that has changed dramatically and today most food is grown using lots of toxic chemicals. In some countries non-organic food is called 'conventional' although this name may mislead some people to believe that this is the way food has always been grown. Furthermore, GMO (genetically modified organisms) have been introduced into our non-organic food supply. The best way to avoid chemicals and GMOs is to buy only organically grown food. If organic food is not available or affordable, you should at least know which non-organic foods are not GMO and contain the lowest residues of toxic chemicals.

Levels of chemical residues in non-organic produce

highest chemical residue levels in fruit
apples, peaches, nectarines, strawberries, grapes, blueberries, pears, raspberries, tangerines

Highest chemical residue levels in vegetables:

Celery, spinach, sweet bell peppers, cucumbers, cherry tomatoes, snap peas, potatoes, hot peppers, lettuce, kale, collard greens, green beans

lowest toxin residue levels in vegetables:

Asparagus, cabbage, sweet peas, carrots, mushrooms

lowest toxin residue levels in fruit:

Pineapples, avocados, watermelons, mangoes, papayas, kiwi, grapefruit, cantaloupe

Plant based non-organic foods that may contain GMO

Non-organic crops that **may** contain GMO are:
Corn, rice, wheat, potatoes, soy, Hawaiian papaya, Arctic apples, sugar-beets, canola, cotton, alfalfa, sorghum,

Notes:

1. As sprouts are an important ingredient in the balanced smoothie, I recommend you try to buy only organic sprouts or grow them yourself.

2. **This list is subject to change as new GMO foods are being continuously approved and released into the market and in most states there is no requirement to label them as such.**

SMOOTHIE INGREDIENTS INFORMATION

The following sections provide detailed information about the ingredients mentioned in this book. The ingredients appear under these categories

Leafy Greens

Leafy Greens – Introduction

Green leafy vegetables constitute a major and essential part of the balanced smoothie recipe. A wide range of leafy green vegetables are available varying with geographical location. The darker the color – the higher concentration of chlorophyll Chlorophylls are a group of green plant pigments that play a central role in photosynthesis, a process involving the conversion of carbon dioxide and water to carbohydrates such as sugars using the sun's light as the source of energy. Chlorophyll is similar in its molecular structure to hemoglobin with the main difference being that hemoglobin is built around iron (Fe), whereas chlorophyll is built around magnesium (Mg). The main function of hemoglobin is to enable red blood cells transport oxygen from the lungs to all parts of the body. Therefore, it is thought that an adequate consumption of dark green leafy vegetable may assist the body in synthesizing hemoglobin. Chlorophyll has been shown in scientific research to decrease colon cancer risk associated with consumption of red meat and exposure to aflatoxin produced by molds found on many types of nuts, grains and dried fruits.

Most dark green leafy vegetables also contain lutein and Zeaxanthin, two powerful antioxidants found in high concentrations in the lens, retina, and macula of the human eye and thought to be crucial to support healthy eyes.

Green leafy vegetables are also high in nitrates, which that are converted into nitric oxide in the body. Nitric oxide, helps dilate blood vessels, improve blood flow and lower blood pressure. Consumption of leafy green vegetables has been shown to contribute to cardiovascular health.

Lowering blood pressure may also contribute to healthy eyes by helping reduce glaucoma risk. People who consumed the most nitrate from leafy green vegetables had a 21 percent lower risk of open-angle glaucoma. Those who ate the most leafy greens were 48 percent less likely to develop para-central glaucoma, which is particularly associated with blood flow

The best form of green leaves is often nicknamed 'baby'. For example, 'baby' spinach leaves. The baby leaves are younger, smaller, more tender, have a nicer flavor, are easier to blend and most importantly more nutrient dense.

Warnings:

1. High oxalate content may increase the risk of formation of kidney and gallbladder stones in people who are predisposed to this condition. If you suffer from or are at risk of formation of kidney and gallbladder stones don't use high oxalate greens such as spinach, beet greens, okra, leeks, collard greens, kale, celery, chard, zucchini, parsley, rhubarb. You should consult your health practitioner regarding foods

that may not be suitable for you and choose your smoothie ingredients accordingly.

2. The so called 'conventional' (a term used for non-organic) leafy greens usually contain a substantial amount of herbicides, pesticides and fungicides. It is best to get fresh organic leafy green vegetables.

Leafy Green vegetables for smoothies

The following green leafy vegetables are widely available and can be used in smoothies:

- **Kale**
- **Spinach**
- **Chard (Silver-beet)**
- **Collard greens**
- **Beet Greens**
- **Sweet Potato leaves**
- **Bok Choy**
- **Watercress**
- **Coriander greens (Cilantro)**
- **Parsley**
- **Basil**

Kale

Among the green leafy vegetables kale stands out due to its high nutrient concentration and its anti-inflammatory power. Kale is a nutrient dense food packed with vitamins A, C, K, and minerals magnesium, manganese, iron, calcium and potassium. It also contains essential Omega fatty acids with a good ratio of Omega 3 to 6 of. It contains the phytonutrients indole-3-carbinol that helps in DNA cell repair and in slowing the growth of cancer cells. It also contains sulforaphane that helps protect against bladder, prostate and colon cancers. It contains the antioxidants lutein and Zeaxanthin that help maintain healthy eyes. Kale has a range of important flavonoids including kaempferol and quercetin that may also play an important role in prevention of cancer.

Warning:

High oxalate content may increase the risk of formation of kidney and gallbladder stones in people who are predisposed to this condition.

Spinach

Spinach is rich in fiber, vitamins, minerals and important flavonoids and antioxidants. It is a good source of vitamins A, C, K and Folate and also contains the minerals magnesium, manganese, iron, calcium and potassium. It has been shown to help muscles utilize oxygen more efficiently. On the down side spinach contains oxalic acid that can bind iron and calcium and reduce their absorption.

Warning:

High oxalate content may increase the risk of formation of kidney and gallbladder stones in people who are predisposed to this condition.

Chard

Chard, is also called rainbow chard due to a range of white, yellow, red, orange and purple stalks in each bunch. Other names include Swiss chard, silver-beet, perpetual spinach, spinach beet, crab beet, bright lights, sea-kale beet, and mangold. It is a dark leafy vegetable, packed with nutrients including fiber, vitamins A, C and K. Minerals include lots of iron and also potassium, manganese, magnesium, copper. It also contains at least 13 different polyphenol antioxidants that help reduce inflammation, protect the cardiovascular system and regulate blood sugar levels. The colored parts of the chard have the highest amounts of polyphenols, so don't throw the stalks away. Scrub well, chop into small bits and use when blending your smoothies.

Warning:

High oxalate content may increase the risk of formation of kidney and gallbladder stones in people who are predisposed to this condition.

Collard greens

Collard greens are a nutrient dense food that belongs to the cruciferous vegetables family and a close genetic relative of the kale and the wild cabbage. Similarly, they are rich in vitamins A, C and K,

B6, riboflavin, Folate, manganese, calcium, magnesium, and iron. Four glucosinolates found in collard greens are glucoraphanin, sinigrin, gluconasturtiin, and glucotropaeolin may help the body detoxify, reduce inflammation and the risk of cancer.

Warning:

High oxalate content may increase the risk of formation of kidney and gallbladder stones in people who are predisposed to this condition.

Beet greens

Beet greens are a nutrient dense nutrient dense food with nutrients that may boost the immune system, support brain function and bone health. Beet greens are rich in fiber, vitamin A, K, B6, magnesium, potassium, copper, and manganese and also contain phosphorus, and zinc and a range of antioxidants.

Warning:

High oxalate content may increase the risk of formation of kidney and gallbladder stones in people who are predisposed to this condition.

Bok Choy

Bok Choy is a cruciferous vegetable cultivated in China for centuries. Bok Choy is a good source for vitamins A, C, K, Folate and B6 and is rich in the minerals magnesium, calcium, potassium, manganese, phosphorus and iron.

Bok Choy is also rich in the antioxidant beta carotene that may help support eye health and a range of other phytonutrients including thiocyanates, lutein, Zeaxanthin, isothiocyanates, and sulforaphane. These are anti-inflammatory. sulforaphane found in bok choy and other cruciferous vegetables may help in preventing cancer, and also in detoxifying the body and supporting kidney health.

Warning:

High oxalate content may increase the risk of formation of kidney and gallbladder stones in people who are predisposed to this condition.

Sweet potato leaves

Watercress Sweet potato (also called batata) leaves are a nutrient dense food rich in dietary fiber, vitamins, minerals, antioxidants, and essential fatty acids including vitamin E (Alpha Tocopherol), A, K, Niacin, Thiamine, Riboflavin, Vitamin B6, Folate, and the minerals Magnesium, Potassium, Manganese and Phosphorus.

Sweet potato leaves may help strengthen immune function, reduce oxidative stress and free radical damage, decrease cardiovascular disease risk, and even help suppress cancer cell growth.

Warning:

High oxalate content may increase the risk of formation of kidney and gallbladder stones in people who are predisposed to this condition.

Watercress

Watercress is a nutrient dense food member of the cabbage or cruciferous veggie family. It contains a range of potent anti-inflammatory phyto-nutrients, is rich in calcium, iron, zinc, potassium and magnesium, vitamins C, A, E and K and several B vitamins, including Folate

Watercress also contains two antioxidants, lutein and Zeaxanthin that are essential for eye health and prevention of cataracts.

Watercress has been shown to reduce damage associated with diabetes and may help improve blood lipid profile. Several studies have shown that a compound called phenylethyl isothiocyanate, found in watercress may suppress cancer cell development by interfering with their signaling capabilities.

Warning:

High oxalate content may increase the risk of formation of kidney and gallbladder stones in people who are predisposed to this condition.

Coriander greens (Cilantro)

Parsley Coriander greens, also called Cilantro is a nutrient dense food rich in many important nutrients. It contains vitamins A, K, and C (in small amounts), K and Folate (B9) as well as the minerals potassium and manganese as well as the antioxidants beta-carotene, beta-cryptoxanthin, lutein and Zeaxanthin that are so important for maintaining eye health. Coriander has been found to have antimicrobial properties as well as lead chelating properties that may help in detoxifying the body of heavy metals.

Warning:

High oxalate content may increase the risk of formation of

kidney and gallbladder stones in people who are predisposed to this condition.

Note:

Use as a garnish in smaller amounts - you only need a few leaves to enhance the flavor of green smoothies.

Parsley

Parsley has laxative and diuretic properties. is a source for vitamins A, C and K. In various studies parsley has been shown to have anti-viral and anti-bacterial properties. It also been shown to have liver protective properties. A substance called apigenin found in parsley and celery was found to exhibit anti-cancer activity. Myricetin, a flavonol found in parsley has been shown to have chemo-preventive effects that may help prevent skin cancer. Myricetin may also help lower insulin resistance, and thus help lower blood sugar levels and help prevent diabetes.

Warning:

High oxalate content may increase the risk of formation of kidney and gallbladder stones in people who are predisposed to this condition.

Note:

Use as a garnish in smaller amounts – you only need a few leaves to enhance the flavor of green smoothies.

Basil

Basil is a fragrant green herb related to peppermint and used for seasoning in Asian and African cuisine.

Basil is very rich in vitamin K and also provides vitamins A, C and Folate in modest amounts. It also contains the minerals manganese, copper, calcium, magnesium and manganese. Basil also contains the flavonoids orientin and vicenin that have been shown to have antioxidant activity.

Basil's nice aroma comes from aromatic oil content including limonene, sabinene, myrcene, estragole, linalool, cineole, and eugenol. These have been shown to have anti-bacterial activity against a range of bacteria including several antibiotic resistant strains.

Note:

Use as a garnish in smaller amounts – you only need a few leaves to enhance the flavor of green smoothies.

Mint

Mint leaves have been used since ancient times as a garnish and in traditional medicine Mint tea is used a refreshing cooling summer drink. It has antioxidant, anti-inflammatory, antibacterial properties and may also help induce sweating. Mint is used in traditional medicine to help alleviate digestive disorders, and help decongest the nasal passages and airways. Mint is used in toothpastes to improve oral health and freshen the mouth.

Other vegetables for smoothies

Introduction

There are many non-leafy vegetables you can use in your balanced smoothies. This section will focus on several great vegetables that are excellent sources of essential nutrients, widely available (in season), reasonably affordable, provide a range of colors (green, yellow, white, orange, red) and flavors (sweet, sour, bitter, salty, pungent).Organic non-GMO vegetables are recommended where possible and affordable. Using pickled vegetables is also a great option that will give your digestive system probiotic support. The easiest veggies to pickle are cabbage and cucumber but you can also pickle beetroot and capsicum (see section on pickling).

Warning:

Scientists believe that a family of compounds called glycoalkaloids contained in Nightshade vegetables, may contribute to pain and inflammation in some people. Nightshades belong to the Solanaceae family which includes very popular vegetables including tomatoes, potatoes, peppers, and eggplant. Other plants that are not nightshades also contain these alkaloids. These include blueberries, huckleberries, goji berries and others. If you are suffering from an inflammation type condition (e.g. arthritis, irritable bower syndrome etc.) you should consult your health practitioner regarding foods that may not be suitable for you and choose your smoothie ingredients accordingly.

Tomatoes

Tomatoes offer a wide variety of nutrients including antioxidants, fiber, significant amounts of vitamins A, C and K, and also vitamins E, B6, thiamine, niacin, Folate, good amounts of the minerals potassium and manganese and also some magnesium, phosphorus, and copper.

One of antioxidants contained in tomatoes is lycopene, a carotene and carotenoid pigment that gives the tomato its bright red color. Scientific studies have shown that lycopene may provide some benefit in reducing the risk of various types of cancer, cardiovascular disease (CVD), diabetes and benign prostate hyperplasia (BPH), as well as help in preventing osteoporosis and maintaining bone health. Studies have shown that the availability of lycopene increases significantly by cooking tomatoes and/or crushing them and mixing with olive oil. Therefore, to get the full nutritional benefit of the tomatoes it is recommended to add a teaspoon of olive oil to your smoothie and mix it well. If you are using a commercial tomato puree, it is best to try to get an organic brand with no added salt or one that contains sea salt.

Warning:

Tomatoes are a very popular vegetable that belong to the Nightshade family. As mentioned above there are various types of inflammation that may be aggravated by consuming nightshades.

Sweet capsicums / Bell peppers

Sweet capsicums come in several varieties including red, orange and green. Capsicums add flavor and color to the smoothies yet contain only moderate amounts of sugar.

The red variety is the sweetest and is rich in vitamins A, C, B6 and K, the mineral potassium and fiber. Bell peppers also contain several antioxidants called carotenoids (lycopene, beta-carotene and Zeaxanthin).

Beetroot

Beetroot is a nutrient dense nutrient dense food high in vitamins including Folate and vitamin C, fiber and essential minerals including potassium, manganese, magnesium, iron, copper and phosphorus.

Beetroot is rich in antioxidants including carotenoids lutein and Zeaxanthin and the flavonoid Anthocyanins Betanin and vulgaxanthin, two powerful antioxidants found in beetroot are anti-inflammatory, and support detoxification.

Beetroot may help in lowering blood pressure, protecting the liver against chemical toxicity, helping prevent and fight cancer and inflammation, increasing stamina, and supporting detoxification. Research has shown that beetroot extract reduced tumor formations in animal models.

Beetroot high nitrate content may help protect blood vessels and enhance exercise performance.

Beetroots can also be pickled (see section on pickling).

Cautions:

1. Beet roots have a very high sugar content equaling that of many sweet fruits, so should be eaten in moderation.

2. As the name implies beet roots grow underground and as such are susceptible to a range of bugs including worms and maggots that dig into the root and feast on it. For this reason, I advise against eating any type of root vegetable in its raw form. I suggest you peel off the skins and then boil several beet roots and store them in the fridge. The boiled beetroots can be stored in the fridge for a few days or frozen in the freezer and later defrosted. Another great way to use cooked beet roots is to cook, slice and then preserve them using salt, vinegar, water and spices. You can then use several thin slices of cooked beet root by adding them to the vegetables in the blender.

Celery

Celery is rich in vitamin K and antioxidants and anti-inflammatory phytonutrients that include dihydrostilbenoids and furanocoumarins like bergapten and psoralen. It also contains vitamins A, C and Folate It provides the minerals potassium and magnesium and dietary fiber. Celery contains a flavonoid called luteolin that has some anti-cancer properties and a phytonutrient called phthalides that has a relaxing effect on artery walls and may help increase blood flow and reduce blood pressure. However, most of the research has been done on celery seed extracts and not on the celery stalk itself and not enough scientific evidence is available on the overall impact of the celery stalk on people with elevated blood pressure.

Warning:

Some people may be allergic to celery and may even have severe allergic reactions when consuming this vegetable. Make sure you are not allergic to celery before incorporating into your smoothie.

Cucumber

Cucumbers are very hydrating and cooling with a high water content of 95 percent. They have anti-inflammatory properties and contain modest amounts of minerals such as magnesium and polyphenols called lignans, that are believed to lower the risk of breast, prostate, uterine, and ovarian cancers.

Cucumbers also contain fisetin – an anti-inflammatory believed to help support brain health. Cucumber peels contain polyphenols and flavonoids that have been shown to alleviate diabetes in animal models.

Cucumbers can be pickled by a process called lactic fermentation. Using pickled cucumbers in your smoothie can give your digestive system a probiotic boost.

Cabbage

Cabbage is rich in vitamin K, that plays a role in bone health and brain health. Cabbage is also rich in vitamins C, thiamine (B1), pyridoxine (B6), and pantothenic acid (B5), Folate, and provides reasonable amounts of the minerals manganese, iron, magnesium, phosphorus, calcium and potassium.

Cabbage is rich in antioxidants including sulforaphane, thiocyanates, lutein, Zeaxanthin and isothiocyanates that may help prevent various types of cancer and reduce "bad cholesterol" levels. Cabbage also provides good amounts of fiber. Red cabbage is rich in Anthocyanins polyphenols – powerful antioxidants that give it its color. Cabbage is rich in glucosinolates are that break down into indoles, sulforaphane and other phytonutrients that may help prevent cancer.

Cabbage can be pickled by a process called lactic fermentation. Using pickled cabbage in your smoothie can give your digestive system a probiotic boost.

Onion

Onion has been used as a food and medicine for thousands of years and is even mentioned in the bible. It is one of the most important culinary plants worldwide.

Onion is rich in very high in polyphenols, flavonoids including quercetin – a powerful antioxidant.

Onion has antibacterial, anti-fungal, anti-inflammatory, antioxidant and immune boosting properties. It has been shown to help prevent cancer and diabetes and help lower cholesterol and blood pressure levels. It may also help improve bone density.

Fennel bulb

Fennel is pungent and warm in nature and has according to traditional medicine may help regulate the energy flow of the liver and digestive system channels. It may help alleviate cold, pain, flatulence, indigestion, reduced appetite, and menstrual pain. Fennel is rich in vitamin C and also in anethole an organic compound found in fennel essential oil that may help prevent cancer. Fennel essential oil has been shown to have anti-clotting and relaxant effect on blood vessels.

Fruit

Introduction

- Fruit are an excellent source of antioxidants, vitamins, enzymes and fiber.

- Most fruit are high in sugars, including fructose, and should eaten in small quantities. Avocados, Lemons and limes are nutrient dense citrus fruits that are very low on sugar.

- In many cases the skin of the fruit has the highest amount of antioxidants and fiber .Ripe fruit has higher concentration of nutrients than unripe fruit and is easier to digest.

- Fruit seeds are very rich in phytonutrients and can be blended too. Some examples are pawpaw seeds, apple seeds, citrus seeds and so on.

- Citrus peel is loaded with antioxidants, vitamins, minerals and fiber. Use only organic non waxed citrus peel.

- Berries in general are delicious nutrient dense foods that are very high in antioxidants and relatively low on sugar. Berries may help fight inflammation and reduce the risk of cancer, cardiovascular disease and eye disease. Antioxidant content is measured and quantified in the lab using "Oxygen Radical Absorbency Capacity" (ORAC). Some of the highest on the ORAC scale are:

Elderberries – 14,697 mean ORAC Score

Wild Blueberries – 9621 mean ORAC Score

Cranberries – 9,090 mean ORAC Score

Blackberries – 5,905 mean ORAC Score

Blueberries – 4669 mean ORAC Score

Cherries – 3747 ORAC Score

Goji berries (wolfberries) – 3290 mean ORAC Score

Blueberries

Blueberries are a nutrient dense food and a staple of the native American diet. Blueberries are high in vitamins A and K and in the minerals potassium and phosphorous. They also contain a range of other vitamins and minerals in smaller quantities. Blueberries contain a wide range of antioxidants including Anthocyanins that give the blueberries their blue color. The high antioxidant content in blueberries may help in reducing inflammation, cancer risk and cardiovascular and diabetes risk factors and also help in improving eye health and preventing eye disease.

Goji Berries

Goji berries are a nutrient dense food, that has been used in Traditional Chinese Medicine (TCM) and cuisine for millennia. goji berries are high in vitamins C, A and

Riboflavin and the minerals iron, copper and potassium. goji berries contain a wide range of antioxidants. The high antioxidant content in goji berries may help in reducing inflammation, cancer risk and cardiovascular and diabetes risk factors. It may also help in improving eye health and preventing eye disease. goji berries have been shown to have chemo-protective properties.

Cranberries

Cranberries are rich in vitamins C, E. Cranberries are rich in other antioxidants including cyanidin, peonidin, and quercetin, oligomeric proanthocyanidins and anthocyanidin flavonoids. Cranberries are also rich and in fiber.

Up to 60% percent of women experience some type of urinary infection at some point in their life. Cranberries may help prevent recurrent infections and even resolve some urinary tract infections by inhibiting bacterial adhesion to bladder and urethra walls. Cranberries may also help prevent some types of cancer.

Warning:

High oxalic acid content may lead to formation of oxalate that may increase the risk of formation of kidney and gallbladder stones in people who are predisposed to this condition.

Note:

Always try to get organic cranberry juice with no added sugar, coloring or preservatives.

Avocado

Avocados are a nutrient dense fatty fruit that is low on complex carbohydrates and very low on sugars in particular with a very low Glycemic index (GI). Avocados are rich in monounsaturated fatty acids (MUFA) that are easily burned for energy. Avocados are low in polyunsaturated fatty acids so do not contribute to omega-3 to omega-6 imbalance. Avocados contains a range of essential nutrients, including the minerals potassium, magnesium, manganese and others and vitamins C, K, Folate, Pantothenic acid, B6 and others in smaller quantities. Avocados high levels of potassium may contribute to balancing out excess sodium in the diet.

Avocados provide many health benefits as they may help optimize cholesterol levels and help reduce the risks of some types of cancer. Avocado seed extract has shown anti-fungal anti-bacterial and anti-worm larva activity. However, avocado seeds are hard to cut and blend and require tough knifes and blenders so I do not recommend using them for the smoothie.

Notes:

1. Try to peel the avocado as close as possible to the skin because the highest concentration of 11 types of carotenoids (a type of antioxidants), are concentrated close to the skin.
2. Avocado fat content may improve absorption of fat soluble phyto-nutrients such as lutein and carotene and pro-vitamin A Carotenoids.

Pomegranate

The pomegranate is a nutrient dense fruit known to man since the dawn of civilization. The easiest way to enjoy the health benefits of pomegranates is to squeeze the juice out and add it to your smoothies. If fresh pomegranates are not available, you can buy bottled organic pomegranate juice. Pomegranates keep well for several months in refrigeration so stocking up on them is also an option.

Pomegranates are rich in vitamin C and K. They also contain the B Vitamins Folate, thiamine, pantothenic acid and pyridoxine. The mineral content includes copper, potassium and manganese. Pomegranates are very rich in antioxidants called polyphenols. Most notably punicalagin, a water soluble phenolic compound that hydrolyzes into a smaller phenolic compound called ellagic acid. Research indicates the antioxidants found in pomegranates may help keep the blood vessels healthy and even help in reducing arterial plaque and preventing oxidation of LDL ("bad") cholesterol and in doing so pomegranates may help reduce the risk of heart disease. Other studies have shown that pomegranates may help in reducing the risk of various cancers and even help in slowing the progression of prostate cancer markers.

Note:

Pomegranates are high in fructose, and therefore should be consumed in moderation. Since they are very rich in antioxidants, small amounts provide substantial health benefits.

Lemon

Lemons are an inexpensive and widely available nutrient dense food. They belong to the citrus fruit family (like limes, oranges and tangerines) and are loaded with vitamins, minerals and antioxidants yet low on sugar. Lemons are very high in vitamin C and also provide reasonable amounts of other vitamins including vitamin A, Folate, thiamine, riboflavin, pantothenic acid, B6 and the minerals iron, magnesium, calcium, potassium, copper and fiber. Lemons are high in antioxidants. Besides vitamins A and C (in the form of ascorbic acid) they are high in ß-carotene, beta-cryptoxanthin, Zeaxanthin and lutein. Lemons are also high in glycosides (a type of flavonoids) called hesperetin and naringenin that work well together with vitamin C.

Like other citrus fruits, lemons contain citric acid, yet despite high levels of ascorbic acid and citric acid lemons may actually aid digestion and help alkalize the body.

Studies have shown that lemons may have cardio-protective properties and also help prevent various type of cancer. Specifically – limonene – a type of limonoid found in the rinds (peels) of citrus fruits is thought to have anti-cancer properties.

The peel is actually the most nutrient rich part of the lemon, containing not only Limonene but also lots of vitamins, minerals, flavonoids and close to 11% fiber. Most are concentrated in the yellow top part of the peel except for fiber that is also concentrated in the white softer part of the peel. Hesperidin, a flavonoid found in citrus peel has been shown to reduce cholesterol and blood pressure and may also have anti-cancer properties.

There are two ways to use the peel. The easiest way is simply to chop up the lemon and blend it together will all other ingredients. The other way is to take a lemon grater micro-plane and grate the thin top yellow part of the peel. Then cut the lemon and squeeze the juice. Finally pour the lemon juice and the grated lemon peel into the blender. This method allows to utilize much of the nutrient content of the peel while reducing the fiber content of the smoothie.

Warning:

Lemon peel and other citrus peel contains high levels of oxalate. High oxalate content may increase the risk of formation of kidney and gallbladder stones in people who are predisposed to this condition. If you suffer from or are at risk of formation of kidney and gallbladder stones don't use high oxalate foods including citrus peel. You should consult your health practitioner regarding foods that may not be suitable for you and choose your smoothie ingredients accordingly.

Caution:

If you want to use the peel make sure that you are using organic NON-waxed lemons. The peel of non-organic lemons may contain lots of chemicals. Even some organic lemons are coated with wax. If you put the peel in a bowl and pour boiling water over it and let it cool you will be able to see whether or not waxy sedimentation forms at the bottom and sides of the bowl.

Lime

Limes are loaded with vitamins, minerals and antioxidants yet low on sugar. Limes are very high in vitamin C and also provide reasonable amounts of other vitamins including vitamin A, Folate, thiamine, riboflavin, pantothenic acid, B6 and the minerals iron, magnesium, calcium, potassium, copper and also fiber (especially in the peel). Limes are high in antioxidants especially Limonoids (such as Limonin Glucoside) which have antioxidant, anti-cancer, antibiotic and detoxifying properties and also work well together with vitamin C. Like other citrus fruits, limes contain citric acid, yet despite high levels of ascorbic acid and citric acid they may actually aid digestion and help alkalize the body.

Limes have been shown to boost conventional medicine in treating parasites, malaria and some types of cancer.

The peel is actually the most nutrient rich part of the lime, containing not only Limonene but also lots of vitamins, minerals, flavonoids and close to 11% fiber. Most are concentrated in the green top part of the peel except for fiber that is also concentrated in the white softer part of the peel. Hesperidin, a flavonoid found in citrus peel has been shown to reduce cholesterol and blood pressure and may also have anti-cancer properties. There are two ways to use the peel. The easiest way is simply to chop up the lime and blend it together will all other ingredients. The other way is to take a lemon grater micro-plane and grate the thin top yellow part of the peel. Then cut the lime and squeeze the juice. Finally pour the juice and the grated peel into the blender. This method allows to utilize much of the nutrient content of the peel while reducing the fiber content of the smoothie.

Warning:

Lime peel and other citrus peel contains high levels of oxalate. High oxalate content may increase the risk of formation of kidney and gallbladder stones in people who are predisposed to this condition. If you suffer from or are at risk of formation of kidney and gallbladder stones don't use high oxalate foods including citrus peel. You should consult your health practitioner regarding foods that may not be suitable for you and choose your smoothie ingredients accordingly.

Caution:

If you want to use the peel make sure that you are using organic NON-waxed lime. The peel of non-organic limes may contain lots of chemicals. Even some organic limes are coated with wax. If you put the peel in a bowl and pour boiling water over it and let it cool you will be able to see whether or not waxy sedimentation forms at the bottom and sides of the bowl.

Papaya (Pawpaw)

Papaya originated in Mexico and Central America where it has been part of traditional diets for centuries. Papaya is a nutrient dense food. It is a good source of antioxidants including flavonoids and carotenes that give it its yellow orange color. It is a very good source of vitamins A, C, E and Folate It also provides small amounts of the vitamins riboflavin, thiamine and niacin and the minerals calcium and iron as well as fiber.

Papaya contains several enzymes, most notably papain, a proteolytic enzyme that helps digest proteins, clean the digestive system and prevent reflux. Papain also has an anti-inflammatory effect on the digestive system and has been used traditionally in folk medicine to help treat ulcers and irritable bowel syndrome (IBS). Papaya may help reduce hypertension, protect the liver against chemical toxicity. Fermented papaya cream has been used traditionally to help treat skin ulceration, wound healing and chapping.

Papaya seeds are small black bitter and pungent seeds that can be found in the center of the papaya fruit. They have been used in folk medicine to help treat parasite and worm infections. So don't throw the seeds away. Store them in a small glass jar in the fridge immersed in apple cider vinegar (ACV). You can then add half to one teaspoon of the pickled papaya seeds to the vegetables in the blender and blend thoroughly to ensure the seeds are ground completely.

Sprouts

Sprouts are a nutrient dense food and an important ingredient in the balanced smoothie. Sprouts are rich in live enzymes, vitamins, minerals, antioxidants, fatty acids and fiber, typically containing about 30 times more nutrients (per weight) than organic vegetables and 100 times more live enzymes (per weight) than organic fruit and vegetables.

Sprouts are widely available. There are many types of sprouts to choose from. The most suitable and readily available sprouts for making smoothies alfalfa sprouts, broccoli sprouts, mung bean sprouts, sunflower sprouts and pea sprouts. If you wish to give your smoothie a zesty or hot flavor you can add small amounts of radish sprouts, onion sprouts or garlic sprouts.

The sprouting process deactivates many of the anti-nutrients that are in the seeds. The minerals in the sprouts are more bio-available as they are bound to proteins. Even non-organic sprouts are usually grown with minimal amount of pesticides and herbicides.

Watercress sprouts are the most nutrient dense of all sprouts. However, they are not as widely available. Watercress sprouts are grown in water and must be soaked separately and washed thoroughly to remove dirt and microbial contamination. They can be stored in water in the refrigerator for 2-3 days and rinsed again before consumption.

Wheat-grass and Barley grass are only used for juicing and should not be used in smoothies.

Broccoli sprouts contain large amounts of glucoraphanin as much as 30 times (per weight) as in the full grown broccoli. Glucoraphanin is a precursor to sulforaphane, a compound shown to help protect against molecular damage caused by carcinogenic chemicals. sulforaphane has also been shown to have anti-inflammatory and anti-oxidant properties. It may help protect the liver and also reduce occurrence of upper respiratory allergic reactions.

You can grow your own sprouts. In warm weather the process takes about a week. I strongly advise against growing sprouts in jars as it is an inconvenient method prone to contamination by mold. To prevent mold from growing in the jars you need to rinse the sprouts several times a day. If mold forms, you have to throw the sprouts away and all your work is lost. The best way to grow sprouts is in flat trays using potting soil as growing media. This also allows you to harvest daily according to your needs.

Cautions:

1. Sprouts must be refrigerated, stored for a short time only and washed well before eating. Due to the way they are grown, sprouts tend to harbor relatively high levels of bacteria. In recent years several serious cases of salmonella poisoning have occurred after eating sprouts. Chinese cooking uses large amounts of bean sprouts. However, they are steamed or stir fried and this greatly reduces the chance of bacterial

infection. When using raw sprouts verify the source, check the due by date, visually inspect for freshness and dispose immediately if you suspect they are not fresh. If you grow the sprouts at home, ensure good sanitation to lower risks of bacterial contamination.

2. Alfalfa sprouts and soy bean sprouts are very popular and widely available. However, GMO (genetically modified) alfalfa and soy is prevalent and has also been contaminating and propagating in non-GMO fields. It is recommended that you verify the source of the sprouts if you wish to avoid consuming GMOs.

Seeds

Introduction

Seeds have a very concentrated nutrient profile. Nutrient density increases significantly when seeds are sprouted. Seeds are relatively hard to digest, therefore, we only use several teaspoons. For example, 1 tsp chia seeds, 1 tsp flaxseeds, 1 tsp nigella seeds and 1 tsp pumpkin seeds.

Caution:

Chia seeds and flaxseeds absorb significant amounts of water and expand. This may block the esophagus and lead to choking. To prevent this, grind the seeds in a seed or coffee grinder and then blend it well with the rest of the ingredients.

Warning:

Some people may be allergic to some seeds and they should probably avoid all seeds

Chia seeds

Chia seeds are loaded with nutrients, may help in reducing cardiovascular risk factors and in regulating blood sugar levels. Originating in South America and Mexico, Chia seeds are now also grown in Australia and available in supermarkets and health food stores worldwide.

The chia seed is high in "complete" protein (i.e. has all essential amino acids in adequate proportions) and in Omega-3 fatty acids that are around 55 percent of its total oil content with a good Omega-3 to Omega-6 fatty acid ratio of about 3:1. The chia seed is rich in B vitamins, minerals including calcium, iron, magnesium, manganese, phosphorus, and zinc, antioxidants and flavonoids.

Research has shown that daily consumption of chia may help lower blood pressure and also lower chronic inflammation.

Chia seeds can absorb water up to 12 times their own weight forming a gel like substance that can be used in making chia based beverages.

Warning:

Some people may be allergic to some seeds and they should probably avoid all seeds.

Caution:

Chia seeds and flaxseeds absorb significant amounts of water and expand. This may block the esophagus and lead to choking. To prevent this, grind the seeds in a seed or coffee grinder and then blend it well with the rest of the ingredients.

Note:

If you add the chia seeds to the blender, they tend to stick and clog the blender, especially under the blades and may be difficult to clean. So after grinding 1 tsp seeds in a seed or coffee grinder and mixing the seeds with water as explained above you may choose to mix the ground flax gel with the prepared smoothie in a bowl.

Flaxseed

Flaxseed (also called linseed) is a relatively inexpensive nutrient dense food with many health benefits. Flaxseed has a good Omega-3 to Omega-6 fatty acid ratio of about 4:1. It also has a good protein profile, although not as "complete" as the chia seed due to lower proportion of the essential amino acid Lysine

Research suggests that consumption of flaxseed may reduce the risk of breast cancer and prostate cancer and also reduce mortality in breast cancer patients. Research also suggests that flaxseed may help in reducing blood pressure, total cholesterol and LDL cholesterol. Flaxseed has two main varieties – brown and golden. In 2009 a GMO contamination has been detected in Canadian flaxseed. The best way to reduce the risk of consuming GMO flax is by purchasing organic flaxseed.

Warning:

Some people may be allergic to some seeds and they should probably avoid all seeds.

Caution:

Chia seeds and flaxseeds absorb significant amounts of water and expand. This may block the esophagus and lead to choking. To prevent this, grind the seeds in a seed or coffee grinder and then blend it well with the rest of the ingredients.

Note:

If you add the flax seeds to the blender, they tend to stick and clog the blender, especially under the blades and may be difficult to clean. So after grinding 1 tsp seeds in a seed or coffee grinder and mixing the seeds with water as explained above you may choose to mix the ground flax gel with the prepared smoothie in a bowl.

Nigella (black cumin) seeds

The seeds of Nigella Sativa have been cultivated in Asia and the middle east since the ancient times. The seeds and oil have been highly regarded by traditional medicine in India, ancient Egypt and the middle east and used to treat a wide range of conditions including bacterial infections, liver and skin disorder, lung and heart disease, diabetes and more.

Research has shown that nigella seeds may have antioxidant, anti-inflammatory, antibacterial, antiviral, anti-fungal and anticancer properties and may also help support the kidneys, liver and digestive system. Thymoquinone found in nigella seeds may support heart and blood vessel health and help normalize blood pressure by improving endothelial dysfunction.

In smoothie making I only use the seeds after grinding them in a seed grinder or coffee grinder.

Warning:

If you are sensitive or allergic to seeds you should not consume nigella seeds

Pumpkin seeds

Pumpkin seeds are rich in minerals including magnesium, manganese, copper, zinc, iron and potassium.

Pumpkin seeds provide "complete" protein with full spectrum essential amino acids.

Studies have indicated pumpkin seeds may help in maintaining prostate health and alleviating postmenopausal symptoms.

Traditional Medicine has used pumpkin seeds together with other ingredients to help in the fight against intestinal parasites.

In smoothie making I only use the seeds after grinding them in a seed grinder or coffee grinder.

Warning:

If you are sensitive or allergic to seeds you should not consume pumpkin seeds

Sunflower seeds

Sunflower seeds are the seeds that grow in the center of the sunflower. Sunflower seeds are a good source of vitamins E, Thiamine (B1), B6 and B3 and the minerals copper, manganese, magnesium, phosphorous and selenium. They also provide moderate amounts of zinc and iron. Sunflower seed are very high in Omega-6 and very low in Omega-3 polyunsaturated fatty acids and may contribute to omega 3 to 6 imbalance that is prevalent in modern diet. Therefore, it is recommended to consume only small amounts. In smoothie making I only use the seeds after grinding them in a seed grinder or coffee grinder.

Warning:

If you are sensitive or allergic to seeds you should not consume sunflower seeds

Sesame seeds

Sesame seeds are a nutrient dense food used for thousands of years in traditional medicine and also for culinary purposes (seeds, paste and oil). Unhulled sesame seeds are very high in several essential minerals including calcium, magnesium, manganese, phosphorous, iron and zinc. They are also high in vitamins Thiamine (B1), Riboflavin (B2), Niacin (B3), and Folate (B9). Sesame seeds contain polyunsaturated fats and monounsaturated fats in similar amounts and also saturated fats. However, these include a high proportion of omega-6 fatty acids and only very small amounts of omega-3 fatty acids and may contribute to Omega-3 to Omega-6 imbalance and should be consumed only in small amounts.

Sesame seeds have antioxidant and anti-inflammatory properties and may help in reducing hypertension, blood glucose and cholesterol levels, and in preventing osteoarthritis and atherosclerosis. Sesamol – a compound found in sesame, has been shown to have chemo-protective and radio-protective properties. Sesamol may help protect the kidneys and liver against toxicity and may help alleviate neuropathic pain in diabetics. Recent studies have indicated that sesame may help in cancer prevention.

There are several varieties of sesame seeds including golden and black seeds. According to traditional Chinese medicine sesame seeds nourish and support the liver and kidneys. The black seeds are especially good for the kidneys.

Hulled sesame paste called Tahini is a popular middle eastern culinary ingredient. However, the shell of the sesame seed contains most of its mineral and antioxidant content. Unhulled sesame paste is now available in many supermarkets and health food stores.

Warning:

If you are sensitive or allergic to seeds you should not consume sesame seeds.

Note:

In smoothie making I only use the seeds after grinding them in a seed grinder or coffee grinder.

Condiments

Salt

The most important condiment is salt. Depending on the quality and quantity of the salt you use it can be a health promoting balancing ingredient in your diet or a slow acting poison. The main component in both good and bad salts is sodium chloride that serves as the main (but not only) source of sodium in our diet. Sodium is an essential ingredient that helps regulate appropriate volume of circulating blood and fluids in tissues and cells. The kidneys regulate sodium levels by excreting excess sodium.

Both high and low sodium levels in the body can be dangerous. High levels are more common and may lead to high blood pressure and other serious health conditions including heart failure, kidney disease and kidney stones, fluid retention, stroke, stomach cancer, thickening of the heart muscle and osteoporosis due to increased loss of calcium. Not getting enough sodium can also be harmful to our health. For example, the body needs sodium to maintain a correct ratio between sodium and potassium that is abundant in many foods we eat including leafy greens, avocados, bananas, mushrooms, potatoes, yogurt, mushrooms. The recommended intake is 6 grams of salt (equivalent to 2300 mg of sodium) per day. The typical western diet contains 2 to

3 times the amount of sodium required to maintain good health. This excess sodium is typically introduced into the diet by consuming processed foods that usually contain added salt.

Getting the right quantity of salt is only half the solution. You also need to ensure you get a good quality salt. Natural sea salt contains many healthy minerals. Commercial "table salt" on the other hand is highly processed, typically produced by heating sea salt to 1200 degrees Fahrenheit and removing all trace minerals. That leaves about 97.5 percent sodium chloride and 2.5 percent of added ingredients that may include anti caking agents, aluminum derivatives (e.g. aluminum silicate), added iodine and even mono sodium glutamate (MSG). These may be toxic to your body. Furthermore, removing all minerals except for sodium chloride leads to biochemical imbalances in your body. Iodine is an essential mineral that has an important role in thyroid health. However, both too little and too much can cause health problems and iodizing the depleted "table salt" may lead to excessive intake.

Celtic sea salt or Himalayan salt are natural, unprocessed and contain a well-balanced variety of trace minerals. For the balanced smoothie I recommend using a good natural sun dried sea salt such as Celtic sea salt or Himalayan salt.

Warning:

Only use natural organic Celtic sea salt or Himalayan salt. NEVER use commercially processed salts including table salt and cooking salt.

Apple Cider Vinegar (ACV)

Vinegar has been discovered thousands of years ago probably due to accidental fermentation of wine to vinegar. It is has been mentioned in the bible and used for millennia in traditional medicine. It can be produced by fermenting various fruit juices including apples, grapes, dates, coconuts, beets and sugary water. We recommend using organic apple cider vinegar (ACV) a nutrient dense food with many health benefits.

ACV contains high concentration of acetic acid that gives it its tart flavor. It also contains citric, lactic, malic, caffeic and gallic acids, vitamins, minerals, amino acids and polyphenols. **ACV** has a very low sugar content as most has been converted to acetic acid during the fermentation process. ACV is used for various external applications including helping fight bad breath, soothing sore throats, alleviating skin itching and more. Research has shown that ACV has significant anti-tumor properties and may also help treat some bacterial skin infections. ACV may also help in controlling blood sugar levels and helping manage type II diabetes and helping with weight loss by reducing absorption of carbohydrates.

Organic unfiltered ACV contains the "mother" (cob-web like sedimentation of yeast, lactic acid bacteria and amino acids at the bottom of the bottle) and has a richer nutritional content.

It is preferable to purchase ACV that comes in a glass bottle as ACV acidity level of around 5% may leach chemicals from plastic bottles.

Note:

Try adding a teaspoon of ACV to your smoothie. You may need to reduce the amount of added lemon juice accordingly so the smoothie doesn't taste too sour.

Chilies

A wide variety of chilies is available, ranging from mild to very hot. Adding a bit of chili to your smoothie can spice it up and counteract the cooling effect of green leafy vegetables. Chilies contain vitamins A and C, K and B6, the mineral potassium and fiber. They get their spicy/hot quality from the substance Capsaicin that helps alleviate pain, improve circulation and reduce the risk of intestinal tumors. It may also help reduce obesity by various mechanisms. Capsaicin has antibacterial and anti-fungal properties against some types of microbes. Chilies have also been shown to help prevent serum lipoprotein oxidation

Pickled Ginger

Ginger root is an aromatic, pungent, spicy herb used in Asian traditional medicine and cuisine for thousands of years and is an essential ingredient in many herbal formulas. Ginger has traditionally been used to warm and strengthen the digestive system, disperse phlegm accumulating in the digestive system and alleviate nausea, colds and pains. In traditional medicine fresh ginger is considered warm in nature whereas dried powdered ginger is considered hot in nature.

Ginger has antioxidant, antibacterial, antiviral, and anti-parasitic properties. Scientific research has found that ginger contains compounds called gingerols that possess strong anti-inflammatory, antioxidant properties that may help in alleviating pain and inflammation associated with rheumatism and arthritis. Another compound found in ginger called 6-shogaol has demonstrated impressive potential to selectively inhibit cancer cells and cancer stem-cells without harming normal cells. Ginger has also shown promise in helping fight type 2 diabetes.

Both the fresh root and the spice made from dried ground root are used in cooking. For smoothies only a small amount of pickled ginger is needed just to add flavor and balance out the cooling effect of the green vegetables. You don't want your smoothie to be too spicy. The pickling process is described in a subsequent section.

Warning:

Ginger roots grow underground and as such are susceptible to a range of bugs including worms and maggots that dig into the root. For this reason, I advise against eating any type of root vegetable in its raw form. They should be peeled and cooked or alternatively peeled, sliced and pickled in vinegar for several days.

Seaweed

Seaweed is a term that describes several species of marine algae found close to ocean beds often along the coast. Edible seaweed is either cultivated or foraged. Most seaweed require cooking but the most popular edible seaweed that does not require cooking is dried Porphyria (Nori) used to wrap sushi rolls.

Nori is rich in manganese and iodine. If eaten in moderation, iodine amounts will not exceed the recommended daily allowance. Nori is also high in beta-carotene, vitamins A, C, Folate and Riboflavin and dietary fiber.

Nori has been shown to have antioxidant properties and anti-cancer activity in lab animal models. It has been shown to have a suppressive effect on radioactive iodine uptake (i.e. it reduces its absorption). Nori may help stabilize cholesterol levels.

Nori does not have a fishy taste and can be added to the smoothies without having a major effect on the overall flavor. The best way to use it is to tear small pieces, soak them in a glass of filtered water, strain and add to other ingredients in the blender.

Note:

If you add the nori to the blender in its dried sheet form you may get chunks sticking to the sides and not mixing well. To prevent this, cut the nori into small pieces first.

Garlic

Garlic has been used as a food and medicine for thousands of years and is even mentioned in the bible. It is one of the most important culinary plants worldwide.

Garlic is rich in oligo-saccharides, selenium, tannins, saponins, phenols, flavonoids, and essential oils

Garlic has antibacterial, anti-fungal, antiviral, anti-parasite anti-inflammatory and immune boosting properties. It has been shown to help prevent cancer and cardiovascular disease, help lower cholesterol and blood pressure levels.

Onion

Onion has been used as a food and medicine for thousands of years and is even mentioned in the bible. It is one of the most important culinary plants worldwide.

Onion is rich in very high in polyphenols, flavonoids including quercetin – a powerful antioxidant.

Onion has antibacterial, anti-fungal, anti-inflammatory, antioxidant and immune boosting properties. It has been shown to help prevent cancer and diabetes and help lower cholesterol and blood pressure levels. It may also help improve bone density.

Oils

Olive oil

Olive oil has been an important culinary ingredient for millennium and is also an important ingredient in the balanced smoothie recipe. You only need about one tablespoon of olive oil per one cup of smoothie.

Olive oil is a good source of a mono-unsaturated Oleic fatty acid (55% to 83%) and the saturated Palmitic fatty acid (7.5% to 20%), and also smaller quantities of polyunsaturated acids. Olive oil is also rich in powerful antioxidants called phenols that may have an anti-inflammatory effect. Olive oil is relatively low in Omega-6 type fatty acids and therefore does not contribute to the omega 3 to omega 6 imbalance created by the consumption of most vegetable oils. Consumption of olive oil may help reduce blood pressure, may reduce the risk of strokes and cardiac events and may also reduce the risk of some types of cancer.

Consumption of olive oil polyphenols has been shown to help reduce the low density lipoprotein (LDL) "bad" cholesterol and may possibly also help increase high density lipoprotein (HDL) "good" cholesterol.

Olive oil may improve absorption of fat soluble phyto-nutrients such as lutein and carotene including pro-vitamin A Carotenoids.

Olive oil is relatively stable in room temperature and keeps well in dark glass bottles without the need for refrigeration.

Cautions:

1. It is recommended you use only cold pressed extra virgin olive oil, preferably organic. Depending on the country you live in you should be mindful of the fact that many imported olive oil products may be fake, adulterated, chemically treated, mixed with GMO soy oil or even unfit for human consumption. If you live in a country that has good quality control measures in place it is advisable to buy locally grown and manufactured olive oil. Always look for recognized stamps of approval on the bottle from recognized certified organizations. However, if you are buying imported oil even stamps of approval and brand names may have been faked. Recent surveys on olive oil imported into the USA report that up to 70% of imports do not live up to acceptable standards.

2. Always buy olive oil that comes in a dark glass bottles, as unfiltered light may make it oxidize and go rancid quicker.

Coconut oil

Coconut oil is extracted from the kernel or meat of coconuts. It contains mostly medium chain saturated fatty acids (MCFA) that make it highly resistant to rancidity and can keep in room temperature for up to 6 months. It is also the most suitable oil for cooking, baking and frying as it has excellent temperature tolerance. The MCFA are easy to digest and cross cell membranes with ease. The fatty acid content in coconut oil includes mostly saturated acids: Lauric acid (52%), Myristic acid (19%), Palmitic acid (11%), Decanoic acid (10%), Caprylic acid (9%). It also contains a small amount of Oleic mono-unsaturated fatty acid (8%) - the same fatty acid found in olive oil.

Coconut oil has been shown to improve cardiovascular performance, elevate "good cholesterol" (HDL), increase cognitive performance in Alzheimer's disease and reduce side effects of chemotherapy. It also has anti-inflammatory properties. In the human body Lauric acid is converted into a monoglyceride called monolaurin that can destroy a range of bacteria, viruses and protozoa. This implies that coconut oil may help support immune function.

Coconut oil fat content may improve absorption of fat soluble phyto-nutrients such as lutein and carotene including pro-vitamin A Carotenoids.

Caution:

It is advisable to buy organic cold pressed extra virgin coconut oil. Other types of coconut oil may be manufactured using various chemical processes and solvents such as hexane.

Note:

Coconut oil is not suitable for most smoothies due to its high melting point around 24° Celsius (76 degrees Fahrenheit). Since in most homes in the west room temperature is around 24° Celsius or lower coconut oil may solidify and create sticky lumps in the smoothie. Therefore, coconut oil is mainly suitable for other types of dishes. However, if your home is warm and the coconut oil is visibly liquid you can certainly use it instead of olive oil. It goes nicely with the sweeter smoothies that have a higher fruit component.

Supplements

Spirulina powder

Spirulina is a blue-green algae type cyanobacteria and has been used by the Aztecs in Mexico hundreds of years ago. It does not require cooking and is very easy to digest and absorb because it does not have cellulose cell walls. It is highly recommended especially for vegans as it is a good source of concentrated complete protein and vitamin B12 that is not available in most vegetable food sources. Spirulina is an amazing nutrient dense food with an unparalleled highly concentrated nutritional profile of amino acids, vitamins, antioxidants, and minerals. spirulina has an impressive protein content of 50 to 70 percent by weight. It contains all of the essential amino acids, and 10 of the 12 non-essential amino acids. It also contains many fatty acids including gamma-linolenic acid (GLA) and sulfolipids. It provides many essential nutrients including, vitamins B12, K and the minerals iodine calcium, iron, magnesium, selenium, manganese, potassium, phosphorous and zinc. It is a source of the carotenoid Zeaxanthin – that is important for maintaining healthy eyes.

Spirulina has been shown to help reduce total cholesterol, "bad" cholesterol (LDL), triglycerides, and help increase "good" cholesterol (HDL). spirulina has also been shown to increase antioxidant capacity, alleviate allergies, help HIV and Hepatitis C patients and possibly reduce risk and help treat some types of cancers. spirulina also shows promise for helping treat type 2 diabetes, heart disease, and neurodegenerative disorders.

Caution:

Always buy spirulina from a reputable source to avoid contamination.

Note:

spirulina powder is very fine and tends to become sticky when added to water so unless your blender is very easy to clean, it is advisable to add the spirulina powder to the smoothie after it has been prepared and served into a cup.

Chlorella powder

Chlorella is a green unicellular fresh-water algae gaining in popularity due to its proven ability to bind to hydrocarbon and metallic toxins such as DDT, PCB, mercury, cadmium and lead and thus assist in detoxification of heavy metals and other toxins. chlorella got its name from the high proportion of chlorophyll, containing more chlorophyll per weight than any other plant. Chlorophyll is good for helping clean the digestive system, liver and blood. Chlorophyll may also reduce the risk of cancer by reducing the availability of carcinogens including a range of synthetic chemicals as well as aflatoxin a carcinogenic mold toxin found on peanuts, corn, various nuts and grains.

Chlorella has very high nutrient density. It contains a fibrous, indigestible outer shell (20%) and inner nutrients (80%). The fibrous material is the component that binds with toxins. It also serves as a pre-biotic substrate supporting the growth of beneficial probiotic bacteria in the intestines. The inner nutrients include 45% protein, 20% fat, 20% carbohydrate, 5% fiber, and 10% minerals and vitamins including vitamin B12. However, to make the nutrients bio-available, the chlorella outer indigestible shell has to be mechanically processed and broken. chlorella is also rich in enzymes that can aid digestion including chlorophyllase and pepsin.

Caution:

Always buy chlorella from a reputable source to avoid contamination.

Note:

chlorella powder is very fine and tends to become sticky when added to water so unless your blender is very easy to clean, it is advisable to add the spirulina powder to the smoothie after it has been prepared and served into a cup.

Wheatgrass powder (dried wheatgrass juice extract)

Wheatgrass juice powder has very high nutrient density with a range of claimed health benefits. It contains a wide range of nutrients including vitamins A, C, K, E, and B1, B2, B6, pantothenic acid, and folic acid. It is rich in minerals in including calcium, magnesium, phosphorous and potassium. It contains 17 amino acids, including 13 essential amino acids required for synthesizing protein. It is also rich in various antioxidants in including superoxide dismutase and beta-carotene.

Wheatgrass is rich in chlorophyll (up to 70%) claimed to help build blood (due to its molecular similarity to hemoglobin) and increase red blood-cell count, help clean the digestive system, liver and blood, help stimulate metabolism and thyroid function. Chlorophyll may also help reduce the risk of cancer by reducing the availability of carcinogens including a range of synthetic chemicals as well as aflatoxin – a carcinogenic mold toxin found on peanuts, corn, various nuts and grains.

Research has shown that wheatgrass juice may provide some benefit in cancer prevention and may also help some patients with leukemia and other cancers by reducing proliferation and inducing cell death (apoptosis). It has may also help reduce hyperlipidemia.

Wheatgrass juice contains a rage of live enzymes. There are claims that the viability of these enzymes is significantly reduced in most wheatgrass powders compared to fresh wheatgrass juice. However, if processed and stored correctly the other nutrients including minerals and vitamins should be viable and comparable to those in the fresh juice.

Warning:

Wheatgrass is grown by sprouting wheat kernels. The US Department of Agriculture (USDA), in its finalized gluten-free label rules, determined that a food is considered gluten-free if it has less than 20 parts per million (PPM) of gluten. USDA scientists added that gluten is found only in the seed kernel and endosperm and not in the stem and leaves of cereal plants. However, arguably there is always a chance of cross contamination or human error in any manufacturing process. Therefore, if you are gluten sensitive or suspect you may be, you may consider exercising caution and avoiding using wheatgrass products. You can get similar nutritional benefits from a range of other plant foods.

Note:

wheatgrass powder is very fine and tends to become sticky when added to water so unless your blender is very easy to clean, it is advisable to add the spirulina powder to the smoothie after it has been prepared and served into a cup.

Barley grass powder (dried barley grass juice extract)

Barley grass juice has very high nutrient density with a range of claimed health benefits. Barley grass is similar to wheatgrass and has similar nutritional properties although less research has been done on barley grass to date.

Barley grass juice contains beta carotene, vitamins B1, B2, B6, pantothenic acid, and folic acid and a range of minerals including potassium, calcium, iron, phosphorus, and magnesium. It also contains chlorophyll, amino acids, enzymes and fiber.

Like wheatgrass, barley grass is rich in chlorophyll (up to 70%) claimed to help build blood (due to its molecular similarity to hemoglobin) and increase red blood-cell count, help clean the digestive system, liver and blood, help stimulate metabolism and thyroid function. Chlorophyll may also help reduce the risk of cancer by reducing the availability of carcinogens including a range of synthetic chemicals as well as aflatoxin a carcinogenic mold toxin found on peanuts, corn, various nuts and grains.

Barley grass has been shown to help reduce symptoms and prolong remission in patients with ulcerative colitis. It has also been shown to reduce hyperlipidemia.

Warning:

Barley grass is grown by sprouting barley kernels. The US Dept of Agriculture (USDA), in its finalized gluten-free label rules, determined that a food is considered gluten-free if it has less than 20 parts per million (PPM) of gluten. USDA scientists added that gluten is found only in the seed kernel and endosperm and not in the stem and leaves of cereal plants. However, arguably there is always a chance of cross contamination or human error in any manufacturing process. Therefore, if you are gluten sensitive or suspect you may be, you may consider exercising caution and avoiding using barley grass products. You can get similar nutritional benefits from a range of other plants based foods.

Note:

Barley grass powder is very fine and tends to become sticky when added to water so unless your blender is very easy to clean, it is may be easier to add the spirulina powder to the smoothie after it has been prepared and served into a cup.

Whey protein concentrate powder

Whey protein is made by concentrating and drying the watery residue of milk separated after the formation of curds during the cheese making process. Whey concentrate is considered an excellent source of full spectrum "complete" protein that is easy to digest, absorb and assimilate. It is widely available and used by many athletes as well as people with weakened digestion including some elderly people and children
Studies has shown that using whey protein concentrate in conjunction with exercise may assist in building and maintaining muscle mass and strength. The best time to have it is 30 minutes before or within 30 minutes after exercising. By adding a scoop of whey protein to your smoothie you get

a complete meal. There are many scoop sized so just use the one provided with the product or follow the instructions on the packaging.

Warning:

If you are sensitive or allergic to dairy products, you should not consume whey protein.

Cautions:

1. Organic whey protein concentrates from the milk of pasture fed (free range) cows is the preferable choice. Non-organic products may be contaminated with antibiotics, hormones, pesticide, herbicide residues, artificial sweeteners and flavorings. Grain fed cows (including organic) produce milk that is lower on several essential nutrients such as Conjugated linoleic acid (CLA).

2. Use protein concentrates NOT protein isolates which are much more processed and stripped of many beneficial nutritional co-factors.

Vegan protein concentrate powder

Vegan protein concentrate is made by concentrating and drying vegetable proteins. Use only full spectrum "complete" protein concentrates. Specifically, it should provide the nine essential amino acids histidine, isoleucine, leucine, Lysine, methionine, phenylalanine, threonine, tryptophan, and valine in correct proportions.

Studies has shown that using protein concentrate in conjunction with exercise may assist in building and maintaining muscle mass and strength. The best time to have it is 30 minutes before or within 30 minutes after exercising.

Note:

By adding a scoop of whey protein to your smoothie you get a complete meal. There are many scoop sized so just use the one provided with the product or follow the instructions on the packaging.

Cautions:

1. Organic protein concentrate is the preferable choice. Non-organic products may be include Genetically modified plants (GMOs) and contaminated with pesticide and herbicide residues, artificial sweeteners and flavorings.

2. Most commercially available protein powders contain soy. Avoid protein powders that contain any soy (both organic or non-organic) as soy contains phytoestrogens and isoflavones that are potent goitrogens that may cause infertility in women and impaired thyroid health and fatigue. Non-fermented soy is believed to have a negative effect on the digestive system. Furthermore, 90% of non-organic soy is GMO and may contain high levels of herbicide and pesticide residues.

3. Use protein concentrates NOT protein isolates which are much more processed and stripped of many beneficial nutritional co-factors.

Spices

Intro

Hundreds of spices are used in cooking and some are also used in traditional herbal medicine. Spices add flavor and also have energetic and nutritional properties. Spices can help balance the flavor, color and energetic properties of the smoothie.

Spices are very concentrated and should be used with care. Use them to enhance and balance the smoothie but do not allow them to take over! The smoothie should not be too spicy, hot, pungent, aromatic etc. The following spices may be used with some of the recipes in this book:

Black Pepper

Dried black pepper powder is a pungent aromatic and hot spice made from dried peppercorns. It is a widely available inexpensive herb used for millennia in cooking and herbal medicine. It helps warm and stimulate the digestive system and may help balance cooling ingredients in some smoothie recipes.

Black pepper has antibacterial, antioxidant, anti-parasitic and anti-inflammatory properties.

In wintertime simple green smoothies may be too cooling for some people, especially those with weaker digestive system, who tend to catch colds easily. Adding black pepper powder in moderation may help spice the smoothie and balance its energetic properties. If you are using pickled ginger as part of your smoothie recipe add black pepper powder with care as the smoothie may become too spicy and hot.

Note:

Studies have shown that using turmeric together with black pepper greatly enhances the absorption of turmeric that is not absorbed effectively on its own.

Cinnamon powder

Dried cinnamon powder is a sweet, pungent and hot spice made from the inner bark of the cinnamon tree. It is a widely available inexpensive herb used for millennia in cooking and herbal medicine. It helps strengthen and warm the kidneys, bladder and digestive system and may help balance cooling ingredients in some smoothie recipes.

Cinnamon has antibacterial, antiviral, antioxidant, anti-parasitic and anti-inflammatory properties. Studies have also shown that cinnamon may help in preventing cancer. cinnamon has been shown to help lower blood sugar levels and increase insulin sensitivity in healthy obese adults.

In wintertime winter simple green smoothies may be too cooling for some people, especially those with weaker digestive system, who tend to catch colds easily. Adding cinnamon powder in moderation may help spice the smoothie and balance its energetic properties. If you are using pickled ginger as part of your smoothie recipe add cinnamon powder with care as the smoothie may become too spicy and hot. The best way to use cinnamon spice powder is to simmer it in a small amount of boiling water, let it cool and then blend it in with the smoothie.

Ginger powder

Dried ginger powder is a pungent and hot spice made from the ginger root. It is a widely available inexpensive herb used for millennia in cooking and herbal medicine. It helps strengthen and warm the digestive system and lungs and may help balance cooling ingredients in some smoothie recipes.

Ginger has antibacterial, antiviral, antioxidant, anti-parasitic and anti-inflammatory properties. Ginger may help relieve joint pain, menstrual pain, headaches and colds. Studies have also shown that ginger may help in preventing cancer.

In wintertime, simple green smoothies may be too cooling for some people, especially those with weaker digestive system and lungs, who may also catch colds easily. Adding ginger powder in moderation may help spice up the smoothie and balance its energetic properties. If you are using pickled ginger as part of your smoothie recipe do not add ginger powder as the smoothie may become too spicy and hot. The best way to use ginger spice powder is to simmer it in a small amount of boiling water, let it cool and then blend it in with the smoothie.

Turmeric powder

Dried turmeric powder is a pungent and warm spice made from the turmeric root. It is a widely available inexpensive herb used for millennia in cooking and herbal medicine. Traditionally it has been used for improving blood and energy flow throughout the body, for relieving pain and supporting liver function. Turmeric is possibly the most studied herb in history. Its yellow color comes from the polyphenol curcumin.

Turmeric has antibacterial, antiviral, antioxidant, anti-parasitic and anti-inflammatory properties. Turmeric may help relieve joint pain, menstrual pain and pain caused by injury. Studies in the animal model have shown that turmeric has several different mechanisms to help prevent cancer, help treat diabetes, help prevent blood clots, help reduce inflammation, help improve endothelial function and even help reduce depressive tendencies.

The best way to use turmeric spice powder is to simmer it in a small amount of boiling water, let it cool and then blend it in with the smoothie.

Note:

The digestive system absorbs only a small percentage of ingested turmeric. Studies have shown that using turmeric together with black pepper greatly enhances the absorption of turmeric.

Cardamom powder

Dried cardamom powder is a pungent and warm spice made from the cardamom pods. It is an herb used for millennia as an ingredient in mild curries, chai tea, Mediterranean coffee and herbal medicine. It helps strengthen and warm the digestive system and may help balance cooling ingredients in some smoothie recipes.

Cardamom has antibacterial, antioxidant properties. Cardamom may help protect the digestive system. Studies have also shown that cardamom may help in preventing cancer.

In wintertime, simple green smoothies may be too cooling for some people, especially those with weaker digestive system. Adding cardamom powder in moderation may help spice up the smoothie and balance its energetic properties. It is not as hot as ginger so may be more suitable for warmer seasons or people with generally warmer constitutions. If you are using pickled ginger as part of your smoothie recipe do not add cardamom powder as the smoothie may become too spicy and hot. The best way to use cardamom spice powder is to simmer it in a small amount of boiling water, let it cool and then blend it in with the smoothie.

Clove powder

Dried cloves powder is a pungent and warm spice. It is a widely available inexpensive herb used for millennia in cooking and herbal medicine. It helps strengthen and warm the digestive system and kidney and may help balance cooling ingredients in some smoothie recipes.

Cloves have antibacterial, anti-fungal, antioxidant, anti-parasitic and anti-inflammatory properties. Cloves may help relieve abdominal pain.

In wintertime simple green smoothies may be too cooling for some people, especially those with weaker digestive system and lungs, who may also catch colds easily. Adding cloves powder in moderation may help spice up the smoothie and balance its energetic properties.

Liquids and juices

Intro

Special liquids and juices can be added to smoothies to boost nutrient content and provide some of the benefits of juicing. In each of the recipes the total amount of liquid has to remain roughly the same. You can use a measuring cup, add the liquids into the cup one by one to make sure you do not exceed the recipe's total liquid content. If needed, top it off with filtered or mineral water to get to recommended amount of liquid.

Green tea

Green tea is a very popular cooling ancient drink with a range of health benefits.

Green tea has anti-toxic, anti-inflammatory and anti-oxidant properties. Green tea may help relieve headaches. Studies have shown green tea may help in the prevention of cardiovascular disease and cancer. Studies have also shown that green tea may help in reducing blood pressure, blood glucose and blood cholesterol levels. Other studies have shown that green tea may have liver protective properties.

Warnings:

1. Tea is a diuretic and should be consumed in moderation

2. Tea bushes tend to absorb relatively high quantities of fluoride from the ground. Fluoride has been shown to have

neurotoxic effects – another reason why it should be consumed in moderation

3.   Non-organic tea is usually sprayed with substantial amounts of pesticides. Organic tea is a better choice.

Black tea

Black tea is a very popular ancient drink with a range of health benefits.

Black tea has anti-toxic, anti-inflammatory, anti-oxidant and anti-bacterial properties. Studies have shown black tea may help in the prevention of cardiovascular disease and cancer and may help in reducing the risk of osteoporosis in the elderly and tooth decay formation in general. Other studies have shown that black tea may have liver protective properties.

Warnings:

1.   Tea is a diuretic and should be consumed in moderation

2.   Tea bushes tend to absorb relatively high quantities of fluoride from the ground. Fluoride has been shown to have neurotoxic effects – another reason why it should be consumed in moderation

3.   Non-organic tea is usually sprayed with substantial amounts of pesticides. Organic tea is a better choice.

Coffee

Coffee is a very popular warming ancient drink with a range of health benefits.

Coffee has anti-inflammatory and anti-oxidant properties. Studies have shown coffee may help in the prevention of cardiovascular disease, diabetes and cancer. Other studies have shown that coffee may have liver protective properties. Studies have also shown that coffee may help in improving concentration and mood.

Warning

1. Non-organic coffee is usually sprayed with substantial amounts of pesticides. Organic coffee is a better choice.
2. Over consumption of coffee may result in hyper-alertness and difficulties in falling asleep. It should not be consumed close to bedtime.

Aloe Vera juice

Aloe Vera has been used by ancient civilizations for millennia. It is now cultivated worldwide for medicinal and cosmetic applications. The sap of the aloe Vera has been used in traditional medicine as a purgative and the gel to treat various skin disorders such as dermatitis, psoriasis, wrinkles and burns and a range of digestive disorders including reflux, constipation and inflammation.

Research has shown aloe Vera gel may possess anti-inflammatory, anti-bacterial, anti-viral properties and has also anti-tumor activity that may help in cancer prevention.

Aloe Vera gel contains vitamins A (beta-carotene), C, E, B12, folic acid, and choline and the minerals calcium, chromium, copper, selenium, magnesium, manganese, potassium, sodium and zinc. It also contains eight enzymes including Bradykinase that may help to reduce skin inflammation (when applied topically) and other enzymes that may help in the breakdown of carbohydrates and fats. It also contains 20 amino acids, including 7 out of the 8 essential amino acids.

Caution:

Some brands of Aloe Vera juice contain preservatives so make sure you are not allergic or sensitive to these additives.

Coconut water

Coconut water is one of nature's most nutrient dense foods - a rich natural source of all main electrolytes the body needs and therefore is the perfect sports drink. Coconut water works very well as the liquid base for the sports smoothie and also works well in fruit based smoothies. It is usually extracted from young, green coconuts. It provides a range of nutrients including natural electrolytes, vitamins (mainly C and B group vitamins), a wide range of minerals (including calcium, magnesium, manganese, potassium, sodium, zinc, copper, phosphorous, iron, selenium), trace elements, enzymes, antioxidants, anti-inflammatory phytonutrients and amino acids. Coconut water is a good source of cytokinins, plant hormones that may help to prevent cancer, blood clots and premature aging. Fresh coconut water is isotonic and sterile and very similar to blood plasma and has been used rarely in emergencies when saline was not available since WWII. You can use coconut water as the liquid base for smoothies.

Fiber

Intro

Fiber and its importance were discussed in preceding section. All whole fruits, vegetables and seeds have some fiber content. This section will mention only foods added specifically to boost fiber content. These include: psyllium seed husks and coconut flour.

Psyllium seed husks

Psyllium seed husks are derived from the seeds of the plant Plantago ovata. Psyllium seed husk are a good source of soluble dietary fiber. Their hygroscopic property allows them to absorb water, expand and become gel like.

Psyllium seed husks are used to relieve constipation, irritable bowel syndrome, and diarrhea and also to maintain regular transit of food via the digestive system by ensuring adequate bulk and water content.

Psyllium seed husks have been shown to relief constipation and mild diarrhea, and help reduce irritable bowel syndrome and pain associated with hemorrhoids. Recent studies have indicated that psyllium seed husk may help in lowering blood cholesterol, sugar and insulin levels, as well as reducing risk of heart disease and diabetes.

Warning:

Psyllium seed husks absorb water and expand. The US Food

and Drug Administration (FDA) has reported that psyllium, and other water-soluble gums, may cause esophageal obstruction, choking, and asphyxiation. Therefore, never use more than a teaspoon and always mix a teaspoon of psyllium seed husks with a glass full of liquids before pouring it into the blender. The suggested way of using it is to mix a teaspoon with the smoothie liquids and let is stand for a few minutes. You may have to stir it a few times. You then pour the solution into the blender and add veggies and fruit as described in the section on how to make the balanced smoothie. This will also prevent forming of lumpy smoothies.

Coconut flour

Coconut flour is very high on soluble and non-soluble fibers (58%). Its fiber content is 5 to 10 times higher than that of all other flours. It is also a good source of saturated fats similar to those in coconut oil (14%), protein (19%) and carbohydrates. It is made from dried and ground coconut meat. Therefore, it is gluten free and hypo-allergenic. You can add 1-2 teaspoons of coconut flour to your smoothie to increase the fiber content and make the smoothie thicker.

Warning:

Coconut flour may absorb water and expand and may cause esophageal obstruction, choking, and asphyxiation.

Therefore, the suggested way of using it is to mix a spoon of coconut flour in the smoothie liquids and let is stand for a few minutes. You may have to stir it a few times. You then pour the liquids into the blender and add veggies and fruit as described in the section on how to make the balanced smoothie.

Other ingredients

Stevia

Stevia is a sugar free natural sweetener extracted from the leaves of the plant Stevia rebaudiana. Stevia does not cause a rise in blood sugar levels. It is widely available as a liquid concentrate, powder and tablets as well as ground dried stevia leaves. Only a few drops or a pinch of stevia powder is required to sweeten a cup of tea, a desert or a smoothie.

The active compounds that gives stevia its sweetness are steviol glycosides. Some of these glycosides are somewhat bitter sweet.

Research has shown that stevia may help in lowering blood sugar and blood pressure levels and in increasing insulin sensitivity.

Caution:

Although stevia is natural, some extraction and powdering processes use chemical solvents. Try to get stevia that has been extracted using a water extraction process.

Note:

Stevia can be used sweeten up your smoothie without adding fruit.

Raw-cocoa powder

Raw cocoa powder is a nutrient dense food made by grinding fermented cacao beans. It has been cultivated in South

America for millennia and is now grown in Africa as well. Cocoa is rich in the minerals magnesium, iron, potassium, zinc, copper, manganese and provides moderate amounts of calcium and selenium.

Scientific studies have shown that cocoa has anti-inflammatory and antioxidant properties that may be beneficial to the cardiovascular system (heart and blood vessels), brain and nervous system. Some of these benefits may be attributed to its and phenol compounds including catechin and resveratrol – both phenols and powerful antioxidants. Some studies have indicated that cocoa may provide antidepressant and "feel-good" benefits. This may be due to its phenethylamine content. This is an alkaloid neurotransmitter and natural antidepressant also found in the brain. Cocoa may also have the ability increase endorphins levels. These are endogenous "high producing" molecules generated during exercise, sex and when having fun. Cocoa may also help boost levels of the neurotransmitter serotonin. This is the endogenous chemical targeted by SSRI type antidepressants.

Note:

Taste-wise, cocoa is probably more suitable for fruit based sweet smoothies. I don't like the taste cocoa produces when mixed with green leafy vegetables so I don't use it often. Cocoa powder is an essential ingredient in an avocado-cocoa smoothie or coconut-cocoa smoothie.

Cautions:

1. Most cacao products tested by independent labs have identified very high levels of the toxic heavy metals cadmium and lead (frequently exceeding 1 ppm) in most including organic brands. It is thought that the cacao tends to absorb and accumulate these chemicals from its environment and also during the processing of the beans into edible products. From 2019 the EU will ban cacao products with high cadmium levels.

2. It is highly recommended to get organic raw cocoa as other varieties are roasted in high temperatures and alkalized using various chemical processes and/or additives. The processing is intended to decrease the bitterness but it also significantly decreases the level of polyphenols and totally removes anthocyanidin.

ABBREVIATIONS AND CONVERSIONS

Abbreviations

ACV – apple cider vinegar

c – cup

gm – gram

ml – milliliter

oz. – ounce

tsp – teaspoon

GI – Glycemic index

Tbsp – tablespoon

TCM – traditional Chinese medicine

wt. – weight

°F – degree Fahrenheit

°C – degree Celsius

Conversions

1 Tbsp = 3 tsp = 0.5 fl oz.

1/8 cup = 2 Tbsp = 1 fl oz.

1/4 cup = 4 Tbsp = 2 fl oz.

1/3 cup = 5 Tbsp + 1 tsp = 2.65 fl oz

3/8 cup = 6 Tbsp = 3 fl oz.

1/2 cup = 8 Tbsp = 4 fl oz.

5/8 cup = 10 Tbsp = 5 fl oz.

2/3 cup = 10 Tbsp + 2 tsp = 5.3 fl oz.

3/4 cup = 12 Tbsp = 6 fl oz.

7/8 cup = 14 Tbsp = 7 fl oz.

1 cup = 16 Tbsp = 8 fl oz.

1 oz = 28.35 gram

1 ml = 1/1000 of a liter

1 pinch = $\frac{1}{16}$ tsp = $\frac{1}{4}$ gm

1 dash = 2 pinches = $\frac{1}{8}$ tsp = $\frac{1}{2}$ gm

ABOUT THE AUTHOR

Jonathan Halpern has a PhD in Health Sciences. His areas of interest include Well-being, Complementary & Alternative medicine, Nutrition, Diets, Detox, Sleep, Sports medicine, Electromagnetic Fields (EMF) effect on Health.

Blog

http://smoothiesinfo.blogspot.com.au/

Email:

smoothiehelp@gmail.com

Other titles by the author on Amazon:

Electromagnetic Radiation Survival Guide

http://www.amazon.com/Electromagnetic-Radiation-Survival-Guide-Solutions/dp/1499323026

www.ingramcontent.com/pod-product-compliance
Lightning Source LLC
Chambersburg PA
CBHW071152290526
45788CB00001BA/430